HORSE AND
RIDER FITNESS

HORSE AND RIDER FITNESS

The Essential Guide for all Riders

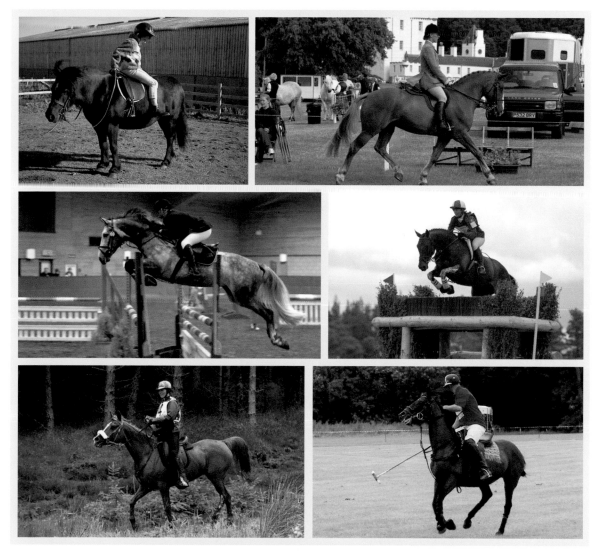

LINDA J PURVES

KENILWORTH PRESS

First published in the UK in 2006
by Kenilworth Press, an imprint of Quiller Publishing Ltd

British Library Cataloguing-in-Publication Data
A catalogue record for this book
is available from the British Library

ISBN 1 872119 96 4
    978 1 872119 96 0

Printed in China

Kenilworth Press

An imprint of Quiller Publishing Ltd
Wykey House, Wykey, Shrewsbury, SY4 1JA
Tel: 01939 261616 Fax: 01939 261606
E-mail: info@quillerbooks.com
Website: www.kenilworthpress.co.uk

Dedication

To my wee man, Sandy, who spent nine months in the womb listening to me tap out this book on the keyboard and then another two in his 'lambing bag' watching me do the same.

To my husband, Andy, for his constant support and endless patience.

ACKNOWLEDGEMENTS

With special thanks to all of the riders who allowed me to photograph them doing their exercises:

Iain and Yvonne Begg
Jackie and Lindsey McDiarmid
Garry Charlish
Liz Armstrong
Joan Austin
Margaret Coward
Michael Goodwill
and to Faraway Riding and Recreation Centre for providing a venue.

Illustrations by Michael Musgrove
Photographs
Show Jumper / Point to Point – John Steven
Dressage / Eventer / Endurance / Le Trec – Peak Photography

FOREWORD

Keeping horses fit is so obviously central to their health and welfare that most books on equine management contain a section on this subject. But even though rider fitness is also important to the welfare of horses it is surprising how little is written about it.

If like me, you have an aversion to gym membership, or if the idea of running endlessly around the roads wearing expensive and ridiculous sporty gear brings you out in a sweat, then fear not! In this excellent book Linda Purves effectively dispels the myth that such exertions are necessary. The book is based on training plans and exercises that are relevant to the equestrian, whether amateur or professional, horse owner or not. To those who are busy juggling their lives around tight schedules which involve work and horses, and who therefore have little time to give to anything else, these plans and exercises will be a real boon.

Linda has kept things simple. Her ideas are realistic and achievable for all riders. What is more, they cost next to nothing in terms of time and money. If all riders spent a little more time on personal fitness it would have a positive impact on their health, riding ability and ultimately will improve the welfare of their horse – so this book deserves a special place on every horseman's bookshelf.

Patrick Print FBHS
Chairman, The British Horse Society

CONTENTS

Acknowledgements   vi

Foreword by Patrick Print FBHS   vii

Introduction   1
  Safety Considerations   2

SECTION ONE – WHAT IS FITNESS?
Chapter One: How Fit are You?   5
  Why Improve Fitness?   10
  The Rider's Muscles – A Quick Guide   11

Chapter Two: Base Fitness Training   15
  Six-Week Training Plan for Horses   16
  Six-Week Training Plan for Riders   17

Chapter Three: The Next Step   24
  What's Next?   28

SECTION TWO – SPORT SPECIFIC TRAINING
Chapter Four: Riding School   31
  The Horse   32
  The Rider   34

Chapter Five: Dressage   45
  The Horse   46
  The Rider   48

Chapter Six: Show Jumping   62
  The Horse   63
  The Rider   64

Chapter Seven: Eventing   74
  The Horse   75
  The Rider   76

Chapter Eight: Endurance   92
  The Horse   93
  The Rider   94

Chapter Nine: Polo   106
  The Horse   107
  The Rider   109

SECTION THREE – FURTHER FITNESS AND FLEXIBILITY TRAINING
Chapter Ten: Injury Prevention   121
  The Importance of Warm-Up   122
  The Importance of Cool Down   126
  Daily Stretches for Riders   127
  Injury Prevention Through Flexibility Training   130
  Advanced Stretches for Riders   133

Chapter Eleven: Onwards and Upwards   142
  Training Using a Heart Rate Monitor   145
  Cross-Training for Fitness   150

Chapter Twelve: Personalise your Programme   152
  Putting It All Together   153
  Update Your Training Record   155

SECTION FOUR – FOOD AND FUN TO FUEL FITNESS
Chapter Thirteen: Do You Eat Like a Horse?   161
  What, When, Why and How Much?   165
  You Can Take a Horse to Water...   168
  Easy Ways to Improve Hydration   170
  Eat Well to Compete Well   171

Chapter Fourteen: Fun Ways to Keep Fit Through Riding   172
  Equercise™ – A Fitness Training Class for Riders 175
  Conclusion   177

Useful Contacts   180

Index   181

INTRODUCTION

I begin this book with a question: are you as fit as your horse? I believe that riders of all levels, whether riding for pleasure or riding competitively, can benefit from taking the time to focus on their own fitness and flexibility as well as that of their horse.

My own experience as a competitive rider, with over twenty years of coaching riders of all ages and abilities, has taught me that both horse and rider must be physically fit if both parties are to achieve their best as a partnership. I find that most riders are prepared to spend huge amounts of time looking after their horses, but spend virtually no time at all looking after themselves. No matter how fit and well your horse is, if you are an unfit rider you become little more than a dead weight in the saddle and, more often than not, a complete hindrance to the natural movement of your horse. New riders soon learn of the tendency for a horse to have a naturally stiff side but sadly the same natural tendency for a rider to be just as one-sided is largely ignored. Time and money are frequently spent on having lessons with all manner of 'experts' in an effort to find the magic formula that will solve all the horse's schooling problems. Invariably, more money is then spent on experimenting with new bits, new saddles and newfangled 'wonder gadgets' that promise to have you performing at Olympic level within twenty minutes! However, when I suggest to those same riders that the key to success is the need to invest time in improving their own fitness and flexibility, I am met with looks of confusion and disbelief.

The aim of this book is to dispel the myth that 'fitness training' involves gym membership, sweaty trainers and Lycra leotards. It need only take a few minutes each day and the majority of the exercises can be incorporated into your daily stable routine. No special equipment is needed, as only everyday yard items are used, so you can turn your stable yard or riding arena into your very own personal training gym. The emphasis is on keeping things simple and relevant to horse riding so that the time you spend exercising off the horse will be of great benefit to both you and your horse once you're back in the saddle.

The first step for all, horses and riders alike, is to achieve a satisfactory level of fitness to allow both parties to enjoy general, non-competitive riding and training. To gain the most from this book I advise all readers to begin with the six-week training plan in Chapter Two – *Base Fitness Training for Riders* – before progressing to Chapter Three – *The Next Step* – and then the more specific exercises for individual disciplines in the following chapters. A number of exercises are repeated in more than one chapter so, to avoid repetitive text, you will be directed to the relevant information where it first appears in the book.

You don't need to be super fit to get started; you don't need to give up hours of precious time; you don't even need to wear matching Lycra as jodhpurs and short boots will do just fine. However, before starting you do need to read through the following safety considerations and, more importantly, you do need to remember that exercising isn't all hard work and it really can be fun!

Safety Considerations

- Always consult your doctor before starting any new exercise programme
- Seek expert advice if you have suffered any serious injuries or are returning to exercise after a long period
- Always warm up gently before exercising as cold muscles are not flexible and you could injure yourself
- Start sensibly as your range of movement will improve over time and avoid forcing your body in any direction that causes discomfort
- Stay relaxed and in control of all movements – keep good posture and remember to breathe
- Stop immediately if any exercise causes pain

WHAT IS FITNESS?

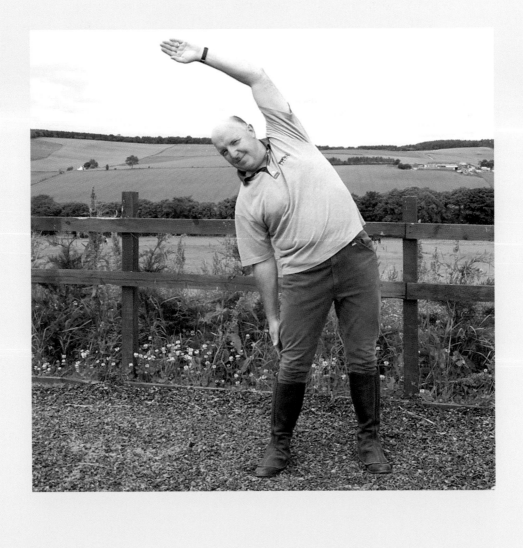

CHAPTER ONE

HOW FIT ARE YOU?

When asked to describe a fit horse, most riders would describe a sleek, muscular competition horse or a horse that is feeling so good about life that it accidentally bucks the rider off as it jumps for sheer joy at every opportunity. The same thought processes usually apply when asked to describe a fit person: Images of lean, finely tuned athletes taking part in Olympic events spring to mind. But fitness is not just about being able to run fast or jump high and it should be everyone's goal to be fit for life, not just fit for sport or competition.

Physical fitness is a part of being a healthy individual. For a person to be described as being in good health they must be free from any illness or injury and also be in a state of both physical and mental well-being. A healthy horse requires exactly the same criteria but would generally be described as being bright-eyed and bushy-tailed.

Physical fitness can be broken down into several components:

- Aerobic endurance
- Anaerobic or muscular endurance
- Speed
- Strength
- Power
- Body composition
- Flexibility

Aerobic Endurance:

Also known as cardiovascular (heart and lungs) or respiratory fitness, aerobic means that energy is produced in the presence of oxygen. Aerobic endurance is dependent upon the cardiovascular system to supply the muscles with oxygen so that they can continue to function for long periods of time. Think of it as the 'Forrest Gump' energy system as it allows you to just keep on going! The type of activities that require high levels of aerobic endurance are generally described as endurance events. Marathon runners or horses competing in long-distance riding events are good examples.

Anaerobic or Muscular Endurance:
Anaerobic means that energy is produced without the presence of oxygen so activities are fuelled by energy stored in the muscles instead. The anaerobic energy system kicks in when the demand for fuel is so great that the aerobic energy system can no longer supply enough oxygen to the working muscles to keep things going. This means that anaerobic endurance is needed for very fast or high intensity exercise lasting only a minute or two. The anaerobic energy system produces a waste product called lactic acid which builds up in the working muscles and quickly forces them to stop – that 'burning' sensation you may have experienced in your muscles! New riders often suffer this muscle discomfort initially as they will tend to use brute strength in place of relaxed muscles to compensate for a lack of balance. Examples of anaerobic endurance in action could be a short-distance sprinter on the athletics track or a horse competing in a jump-off against the clock.

Speed:
Pure speed is perhaps best demonstrated by the 100 metre sprinters on the athletics track and could also be considered an essential component of fitness for racehorses racing over very short distances. However, most equine sports require only an element of speed along with other fitness components such as strength and endurance. For example, a polo pony must be able to travel at high speed to chase the ball but these short bursts of speed are interspersed with many stops and turns throughout the duration of a match.

Strength:
Strength can be defined as the ability of a muscle or muscle group to exert a force. Any ridden horse must have enough strength in his back muscles to carry the weight of the rider and then needs greater degrees of strength to propel itself forwards whilst maintaining balance. An obvious example of human strength could be demonstrated by a weightlifter but in the equine world it is usually the image of a heavy horse pulling a load that depicts strength best. In modern equine sport it could be argued that it is the advanced dressage horse who requires the most strength to perform well.

Power:
Power can be defined as 'explosive' movement or strength in motion. In other words, power is a combination of both strength and speed so perhaps the best example would be to imagine a 100 metre sprinter 'powering' out of the starting blocks. Horses taking part in showjumping and eventing also demonstrate great power as they negotiate courses of jumps, particularly

bounce fences. They have strength to take off and speed to propel them forwards – a powerful combination.

Body Composition:

Body composition is the body's physical make up in terms of fat and muscle (non-fat) tissue. Fat levels above recommended guidelines are undesirable as excess can be detrimental to health and performance. Fat is an essential part of a healthy diet and the body needs a certain amount to function well. However, excess fat is also stored by the body and can lead to certain types of heart disease, high blood-pressure, asthma and diabetes. The body stores fat for survival in case of times of famine or extreme hardship. Arctic explorers and cross-Channel swimmers need to begin their journeys with relatively high body fat reserves as this will soon be used up to fuel their activities and to keep them warm. However, in today's western world the shops are never too far away or closed for long enough that we might face starvation so our bodies no longer require the extra 'back up' for survival. Unfortunately, our bodies still hold on to the excess – just in case! Lean tissue can also be described as lean muscle mass. Contrary to popular belief, body weight is not a prime consideration within the context of body composition as lean muscle tissue weighs more than fat tissue. It is the percentage of body fat compared to lean tissue that is directly related to health and performance.

Flexibility:

Flexibility can be defined as the ability to move a joint through its complete and natural range of movement. Various factors can affect flexibility including the condition of the muscles, tendons and ligaments around the bones that form the joint. Excess body fat in adjacent limbs will also affect the range of movement as will scar tissue from any old injuries in the working muscles.

The benefits of becoming a more flexible rider are many and include:

• Increased body awareness – allowing a better understanding and use of seat and leg aids
• Reduced muscle tension – promoting a more relaxed position in the saddle
• Increased mobility – allowing freer movement with the horse
• Reduced risk of injury, back problems in particular – often caused by tight hamstring muscles and prevalent in horse riders

Not all activities or sports require the participant to possess a high level of all the listed components but for someone to be considered fit for their sport they must be able to meet the demands of that particular activity without placing undue stress on their body. Let's take an average leisure rider, riding three or four times a week, as an example. This rider would need:

- A good level of aerobic endurance
- A high degree of flexibility to be able to sit correctly in the saddle and move with the horse
- A degree of strength, particularly in the core (trunk) muscles in order to maintain a correct riding position
- No real need for muscular endurance
- No need for speed
- No need for power
- Body composition is not of immediate importance (other than health concerns) as people of all shapes and sizes can ride

Now let's look at the leisure rider's horse's needs:

- A good level of aerobic endurance to be able to work mainly in walk and trot
- A good level of strength to be able to carry the rider's weight and to maintain balance
- A good level of flexibility to be able to perform school exercises, to remain balanced through changes of pace and to work over varying terrain
- A degree of anaerobic and muscular endurance to cope with the odd round of jumps or short bursts of speed
- No real need for speed
- No real need for power
- Body composition will have a direct effect on fitness for the job as excess body fat potentially will create breathing difficulties and other health issues

Both rider and horse will then need a greater degree of overall fitness if they wish to progress to more competitive activities and the particular components of fitness needed will vary depending on the event. The key to success is to train specifically for the demands of the chosen sport. It takes time for the body, whether human or equine, to respond to any training and in all cases the only effective way to make improvements is to train progressively over a suitable period of time. To make sure that both parties are fit for a chosen event it is necessary to know what the current level of fitness actually is and what level of fitness will be needed to compete. Only then can a suitable programme of training be put together and an appropriate period of time allowed to achieve the desired results. Someone who finds it difficult to catch their breath after running for a bus would be unwise to enter the London Marathon the following weekend. It would be just as unwise to take a horse from the field after a month or two of relative inactivity and then enter him in the Burghley Horse Trials the following week.

A simple way to gauge your current level of fitness is to try the following eight-hundred-metre (half-mile) walking test which was developed by Merrell footwear. Most people can walk the distance within ten minutes so it is known as the Merrell® Ten Minute Challenge. Walk as fast as you can with reasonable comfort, and time how long it takes you to complete half a mile. It is important to remain in walk and not to jog or run as this would invalidate the test results. Aim to use a reasonably flat piece of ground which you know to be of the correct distance (you could measure a stretch of road in your car) or use your riding arena. If you have a standard 40 by 20 metre (130 by 65 feet) arena you will need to walk six complete laps around the edge, plus go down one more long side and back again, to achieve your eight-hundred-metre (half-mile) target. Compare your time in minutes and seconds against the following chart which is broken down into age groups and is specific to either male or female participants.

> **Note:** always check with your doctor before taking part in any physical activity if you are new to exercise.

Merrell® Ten Minute Challenge – Half-mile Walking Test For Aerobic Fitness

Age	20 - 29	30 - 39	40 - 49	50 - 59	60 +
Women					
High	< 5:37	< 5:55	< 6:17	< 6:40	< 7:07
Above average	5:37 - 6:27	5:55 - 7:00	6:17 - 7:21	6:40 - 7:53	7:07 - 8:31
Average	6:28 - 7:31	7:01 - 8:05	7:22 - 8:45	7:54 - 9:16	8:32 - 10:29
Below average	7:32 - 8:59	8:06 - 10:09	8:46 - 10:29	9:17 - 11:12	10:30 - 12:04
Low	> 9:00	> 10:10	> 10:30	> 11:13	> 12:05
Men					
High	< 5:14	< 5:37	< 5:55	< 6:09	< 6:24
Above average	5:14 - 6:12	5:37 - 6:27	5:55 - 7:00	6:09 - 7:21	6:24 - 7:31
Average	6:13 - 7:21	6:28 - 7:31	7:01 - 8:18	7:22 - 8:45	7:32 - 9:00
Below average	7:22 - 8:31	7:32 - 8:45	8:19 - 9:49	8:46 - 10:09	9:01 - 10:49
Low	> 8:32	> 8:46	> 9:50	> 10:10	> 10:50

Why Improve Fitness?

People who are fit aren't necessarily elite athletes. They are people who have enough energy to get them through their daily activities without feeling excessively tired and they'll also have enough energy left over at the end of routine daily tasks to allow them to take part in other activities away from the workplace or home. In other words, they are fit for life. The American College of Sports Medicine defines fitness as 'The ability to perform moderate to vigorous levels of physical activity without undue fatigue and the capability of maintaining such ability throughout life.'

Unless you are in a position to ride several fit horses a day on a regular basis it is unlikely that the time you spend in the saddle will have any real effect on your actual level of fitness. By improving your general fitness you will have more available energy to get you through your day and therefore more energy left over to enjoy your riding time. By increasing your fitness for riding you will not only be benefiting yourself but also your horse. You will be better placed to help rather than hinder when in the saddle and you will be far better prepared to cope with the physical demands of training without danger of injury to either party. Whether your aim is to ride purely for pleasure or to compete at top level, all riders need to develop a high degree of flexibility to allow them to reach their true potential.

A simple way to test your current level of flexibility is to try the Sit And Reach Test which measures general lower back and hamstring muscle flexibility. This test is not considered an exact science but is used widely at all levels in most sports, although the results are used as a guide only. It's quick and easy to do and the only equipment you need is a measuring tape or ruler and someone to do the measuring for you.

Sit And Reach Test Protocol

> **Important note:** your muscles must be thoroughly warmed up before taking this test

- Sit on the ground with your legs, slightly apart, straight out in front of you
- Make sure your knees are flat to the ground and your ankles are relaxed
- Reach forwards along the floor between your legs by bending from your hips
- Keep good posture in your upper body – avoid folding from your waist or rounding your shoulders
- Continue to reach forwards slowly and then hold still at the furthest point for a count of three – no bouncing or jerking!

• Get someone to measure how far forwards you have managed to reach in relation to your toes
• Three attempts are permitted and the best score is then used as the test result
• Compare your result to the table below to see how you score – note that the distance short of the toes is recorded as well as past the toes

Sit And Reach Test Result	Rating
20 + cm (8 + in) past toes	excellent
10 - 20 cm (4-8in) past toes	very good
0 - 10 cm (0-4in) past toes	above average
toe line	average
0 - 10 cm (0-4in) short of toes	below average
10 + cm (4 + in) short of toes	poor

The result of your flexibility test, along with your eight-hundred-metre (half-mile) walk time, should be kept in a file to begin your own fitness training record. After completing a suitable training programme (at least six weeks of base fitness training) the tests can be repeated to provide a comparison and to chart your progress. Suggested ways to update your file are given in Chapter Twelve.

Achieving and maintaining a satisfactory base level of fitness and flexibility need only take a few minutes out of each day. The following chapters show you how easy it is to turn your yard into your very own personal gym and how, with just a little extra effort each day, you can quickly realise the benefits of becoming a fitter rider.

The Rider's Muscles – A Quick Guide

Biceps:
These are the muscles that form the front of your upper arm; your 'Popeye' muscles! They are your lifting and pulling muscles – they bend your arm from your elbow – so they work each time you pick up and carry a water bucket or shovel a load of muck into a wheelbarrow.

Triceps:
The triceps are the opposing muscles to the biceps so they form the back of your upper arm. They are your pushing muscles – they straighten your

arm at the elbow – so they work each time you muck out, sweep the yard or groom your horse thoroughly.

Pectorals:
The pectorals are your chest muscles and are used mainly when bringing your arm towards or across your body. They are used in the process of grooming, mucking out and sweeping as well as enabling the polo player to take a swing at those awkward under neck shots.

Rhomboids:
The rhomboids are part of your upper back muscles and are found between your shoulder blades. They work each time you correct your posture by pulling your shoulders back to sit taller in the saddle.

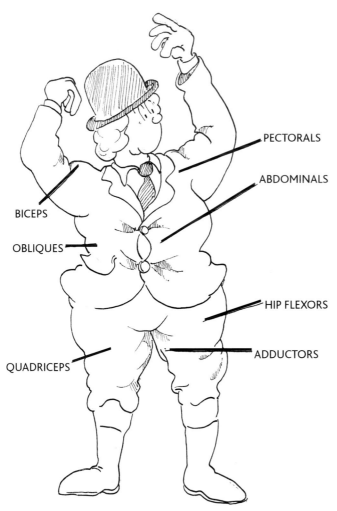

BICEPS

OBLIQUES

QUADRICEPS

PECTORALS

ABDOMINALS

HIP FLEXORS

ADDUCTORS

Latissimus Dorsi:
These are the large muscles that form the bulk of your back and are often referred to as your lats for short. One of their functions is to draw your shoulder downwards and backwards so they work together with the rhomboids to keep you sitting correctly with good posture in the saddle. They also work, along with the biceps, when you're holding on to that pulling horse!

Abdominals:
These are your stomach muscles of which there are many. They form layers around your mid-section and work together to compress your abdomen, rotate your spine and allow you to bend forwards through your waist.

Obliques:
These form part of your abdominal muscles and are found to the side of your trunk.

The obliques along with the other abdominal muscles and the main muscles of the back are collectively known as the core stability muscles. They work together to stabilise your body, keep you in balance in the saddle and allow you to maintain correct, upright posture.

Gluteals:

The gluteal muscles are those of your bottom and are often referred to as your glutes for short. They work to 'open' your hip joint and to take your leg away from your body so they are used to allow you to sit with a 'deep seat' in the saddle. They are also recruited in the process of mounting up and when rising to the trot. Firm glutes are very helpful if you wish to look good in jodhpurs!

Hip Flexors:

These are the muscles that cross over the front of your hip joint where your leg meets your pelvis. As the name suggests, they are responsible for flexing your hip – lifting your leg upwards and forwards. They are used each time you mount up and also when you adjust your stirrup leathers or tighten your girth when in the saddle.

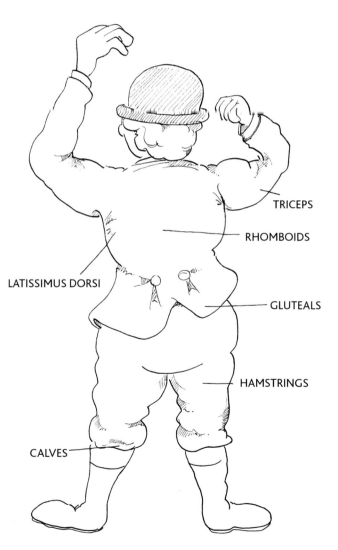

TRICEPS

RHOMBOIDS

LATISSIMUS DORSI

GLUTEALS

HAMSTRINGS

CALVES

Quadriceps:

The quadriceps are the front of thigh muscles and they work to straighten your leg from the knee. They are used to assist in a rising trot but work mainly when riding in a 'forward seat' or jumping position.

Hamstrings:

These are the muscles that form the back of your thigh so they are the opposing group to the quadriceps and therefore work to bend your leg from the knee. The hamstring and quadricep muscles are recruited each time you walk or run, when you mount up from the ground and also when you bend your knees to pick up a heavy load such as a shavings bale.

Adductors:

These are the muscles of your inner thigh. Their main function is to bring your leg towards your body so, as far as riding is concerned, it is far more important that the adductor muscles are able to remain relaxed and flexible, rather than strong, to allow the rider to sit into the saddle. New riders will often experience extreme discomfort in this area as they tend to grip the saddle with their thighs through lack of balance.

Calves:

The calf muscles are found at the back of your lower leg. They work to allow you to raise your heel and go up on your toes so they are in action each time you mount up, particularly from the ground. Flexible calf muscles are very important to the rider as they will allow the heel to drop down in the stirrup and an effective lower leg position to be maintained.

CHAPTER TWO

BASE FITNESS TRAINING

Athletes in a wide range of sports have training programmes that span an entire year. The purpose of such programmes is to allow each individual an opportunity to prepare for the most important event/s in their competition calendar for that season. Each athlete must ensure that they reach optimal fitness for each significant event on that calendar, whether it be a qualifying round or a final. Sadly, it is not physically possible to remain at peak fitness throughout an entire year so it is necessary to schedule for periods of rest and recovery as well as periods of high intensity training.

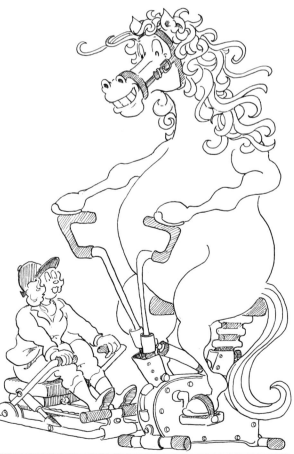

The first phase of training after an end of season rest period is known as base fitness training. This is when the body is slowly prepared for the rigours of more intensive training which will be introduced later in the programme. Without an adequate base level of fitness the risk of injury is particularly high. All too often inexperienced athletes, or people who suddenly decide to get off the couch and get themselves fitter, will rush straight into intensive training and generally do far too much too soon. The physical strain on an unconditioned body will typically result in fatigue and recurring injuries. On top of that, the mental strain of struggling to achieve unrealistic goals will generally lead to extreme demotivation and the individual may simply give up.

Appropriate base fitness training is required for both the horse and the horse rider although, in many cases, the latter is regrettably neglected. The following examples of a six-week base fitness training programme show how to progress both parties from a deconditioned state to a level of fitness that would allow them to safely advance to more specific exercises for their chosen activity.

> **Note:** the following plan is designed for horses who have previously been in work. Young horses require a longer period of slow work in the early stages.

Base Fitness For Horses – Six-Week Training Plan

Week One:
In walk only – three or four rides (hacks) of thirty to forty minutes duration over reasonably flat terrain. Initially, avoid exercising on consecutive days to allow out of condition muscles more recovery time before working again.

Week Two:
In walk only – three or four rides (hacks) of forty to fifty minutes duration. Introduce some gentle hills where possible and / or work occasionally on consecutive days to begin increasing the workload.

Week Three:
Walk and short trots – three or four rides (hacks) of fifty minutes to one hour duration. Where possible, make use of hills (not too steep) – both uphill and downhill in walk only to continue conditioning the muscles. Encourage an active forward-going walk with a contact at all times to help develop top-line muscles. Short trots should be no further than the distance between two telegraph poles and no more than three or four trots in total on each ride. Long stretches of trot on hard surfaces (Tarmac) at this stage could be damaging to the limbs.

Week Four:
Walk and trot – four or five rides (hacks and school work) of forty-five minutes to one hour duration. Introductory school sessions need only be twenty to thirty minutes long and kept simple to avoid over-taxing the muscles at this stage. Work in walk and trot only, concentrating on encouraging correct bend using circles, loops and serpentines, and balance through transitions. Be aware of the importance of riding on the correct trot diagonal to aid symmetry in the horse's body.

On hacks, progressively longer trots should now be encouraged – always warm up in walk before introducing trot – and also include trot on some gradual uphill stretches but avoid pushing the pace beyond the horse's comfort zone (avoid laboured breathing).

Week Five:

Walk, trot, and short canters – aim for five rides (hacks and school work). Ideally, include a mix of three hacks of forty-five minutes to one hour duration and two schooling sessions of twenty to thirty minutes.

Introduce short, steady canters on relatively level terrain when hacking – no more than one or two in total on each ride.

Continue to work in mainly walk and trot when schooling. Short canters can be introduced – be aware of the importance of using both leading legs – but avoid small circles and tight turns which may place too much stress on the working muscles at this stage. Perfect all schooling exercises in trot before progressing to canter.

Week Six:

At this stage the horse should be feeling fit for all light work activities – simple schooling, lessons, light lungeing, hacking out – in walk, trot and canter.

Always allow a minimum of one complete rest day each week and try to vary the routine as much as possible to prevent boredom. The above plan will not necessarily suit all circumstances but the most important thing to remember is that the horse will respond best to a structured timetable, and safe progress can only be made by adopting a step-by-step approach to training. Horses benefit from spending free time in the field (unless on a strict diet!) but, in the case of a permanently stabled horse, walking out in hand should be included as part of each rest day routine.

Base Fitness For Riders – A Six-Week Training Plan

Note: check with your doctor before beginning any new exercise routine.

Tips: build up gradually to a minimum of one hour of exercise (off the horse) each week, whether that is split into three sessions of twenty minutes, four sessions of fifteen minutes, or even six sessions of ten minutes. Always allow your body at least one day of complete recovery each week and initially avoid exercising on consecutive days to allow your body time to adapt to new movements.

Week One:

Begin with two exercise sessions of twenty minutes duration (not including riding time).

Aerobic Endurance Exercises:

Start each session with a walk of about ten minutes around your horse's field. Walk with real purpose and don't shy away from hills as varied terrain will work your muscles, heart and lungs every bit as well as it will your horse's. Use the walk as an opportunity to check the fence or the water trough and why not pick up any litter you find along the way?

Alternatives to walking: yard sweeping / mucking out / grooming thoroughly – any activity that elevates your heart rate and leaves you feeling warm.

See Chapter Ten – *Warm-Up Routines for Riders* – for more detail.

Flexibility Exercises:

> **Tips:** your range of movement will improve over time so start sensibly and avoid forcing your body in any direction that causes discomfort. Stop immediately if any exercise causes pain.

Shoulder Shrugs – to warm up the shoulder joints (*see* pictures 1a and 1b)

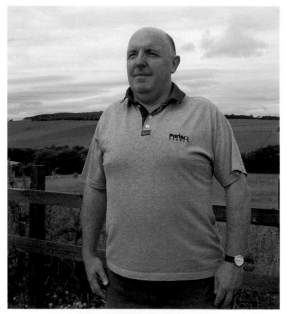

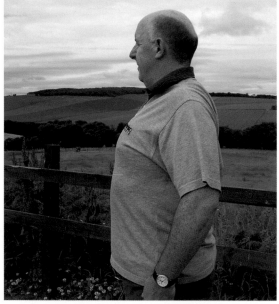

1a Shrug shoulders upwards   *1b Circle shoulders backwards*

Repeat five times.

- Stand with your feet placed hip-width apart and keep a slight bend in your knees
- Shrug both shoulders up towards your ears and then circle them backwards and down again to the starting position
- Keep good posture throughout and move in a slow, controlled manner
- Breathe in as you shrug and out as you relax each time

Arm Circles – to loosen the shoulder joints (*see* pictures 2a, 2b and 2c)

Circle each arm five times.

- Stand with your feet hip-width apart and keep a slight bend in your knees
- Circle your right arm as if swimming backstroke
- Move in a slow, controlled manner and aim for as much movement through your shoulder joint as possible
- Complete five circles with your right arm before changing to repeat the exercise with your left arm
- Keep good posture and breathe normally

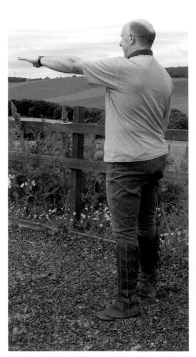 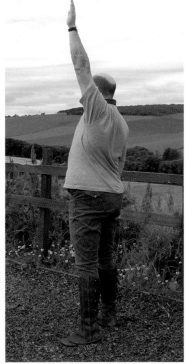 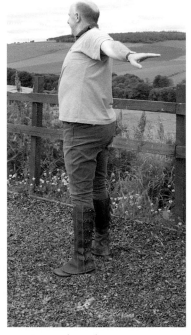

2a Left arm circle   *2b Circle arm backwards*   *2c Backstroke movement*

Side Stretches – to stretch the trunk and arm muscles (*see* pictures 3a, 3b and 3c)

Stretch to each side five times.

- Stand with your feet hip-width apart and relaxed at the knee
- Allow your arms to hang by your sides and then lean over to the right until you feel the stretch down the left side of your body
- Bring your left arm up and over to the right to increase the stretch
- Breathe out as you stretch and hold for a few seconds
- Breathe in as you return to the starting position and then repeat the exercise by leaning over to the other (left) side
- Keep good posture – imagine you have a pane of glass in front of you and behind you as you lean to the side – avoid tilting forwards or backwards.

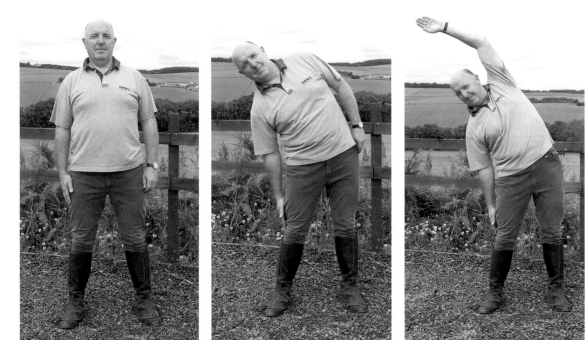

3a Side stretches   *3b Stretch to the right*   *3c Increase the stretch*

Hip Swings – to loosen the hip joints (*see* pictures 4a and 4b)

Swing each leg five times.

- Stand on your left leg (relaxed knee) and lean against something with your left hand for balance
- Lift your right leg, with knee bent, up in front of you as high as you comfortably can

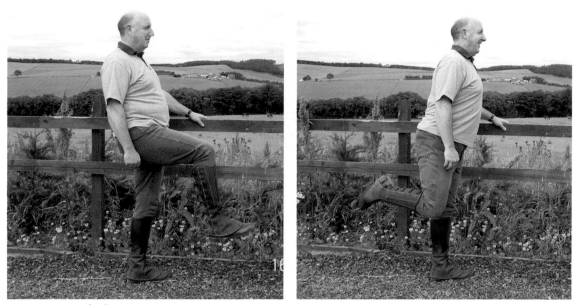

4a Right leg hip swing   *4b Maintain good posture*

- Swing your right leg (gently) backwards behind you – remain upright and keep good posture in your upper body
- Take your time and breathe normally
- Complete five swings with your right leg before changing position to repeat the exercise with your left leg

Week Two:
Aim for three exercise sessions of twenty minutes duration.

Aerobic Endurance Exercises:
Follow last week's programme but add an extra session to make three this week.

It is very important to have warmed up with a brisk walk of at least ten minutes (or alternative exercises) before commencing the flexibility exercises. Your body will now be familiar with the routine so expect the exercises to begin feeling easier than before but take your time and focus on correct technique at all times.

Flexibility Exercises:
Cold muscles are not flexible so they must be warm to prevent potential injury.

Continue with shoulder shrugs / arm circles / side stretches / and hip swings as before.

Week Three:

Aim for three exercise sessions of twenty minutes duration or try increasing to thirty minutes if you feel ready.

Aerobic Endurance Exercises:

Begin each session with a brisk walk of at least ten minutes as before – add an extra five minutes if possible. If you enjoy jogging (not compulsory!) then try adding two or three short jogs on the way round the field.

Flexibility Exercises:

Continue with shoulder shrugs / arm circles / side stretches / hip swings then add –

Trunk Rotation – to loosen the spine (*see* pictures 5a and 5b)

Rotate to each side five times.

- Stand with feet placed hip-width apart and remain relaxed at the knee
- Position the lunge whip (or yard broom) in the small of your back – keep good posture
- Twist through your waist to the right; return to the centre; twist to the left
- Take your time, stay controlled and breathe normally

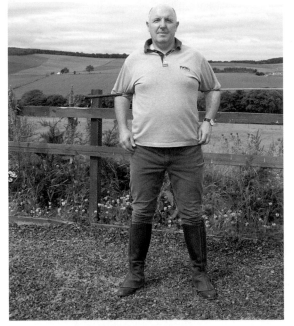

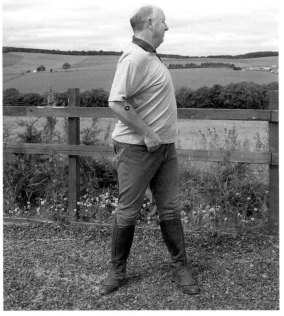

5a Position the lunge whip in the small of your back   *5b Trunk rotation left*

Week Four:

Aim for three exercise sessions of twenty to thirty minutes duration – as last week.

Continue practising the exercises already learned to consolidate your efforts so far.

> **Tips:** try to establish a regular routine so that it becomes habit. For example, Monday, Wednesday, Friday, or Tuesday, Thursday, Saturday would work well.

Week Five:

Aim for three exercise sessions of twenty to thirty minutes duration.

Aerobic Endurance Exercises:

Continue to begin each session with a ten to fifteen minute brisk walk and add a few more short jogs if you enjoy running.

Flexibility Exercises:

Continue with shoulder shrugs / arm circles / side stretches / hip swings / and trunk rotation as last week but increase the repetition of each exercise from five times up to ten times.

> **Tips:** to save time, shoulder shrugs and arm circles could be performed on the move as part of your aerobic exercise warm up.

Week Six:

You should now be feeling fitter and more flexible. Your body is better conditioned and prepared to cope with more specific training, whether that be aerobic fitness, muscle endurance, strength or flexibility training. It is important to have reached this level of fitness before progressing to more demanding training so if you have struggled with any elements of this programme it would be advisable to repeat the exercises for a few more weeks before moving on to the next chapter.

> **Note:** fitness cannot be stored so reaching the end of this six-week programme does not mean that you can now sit back and relax! Continue with these twenty minute sessions on a regular basis to maintain your base level of fitness.

CHAPTER THREE

THE NEXT STEP

Once a solid base level of fitness has been achieved, the next step is to begin training for the more specific demands of your activity. In the case of the leisure rider highlighted in Chapter One, the fitness components most needed are aerobic endurance and flexibility. The simplest, least time-consuming, and arguably the most effective way to improve cardiovascular fitness is to begin a jogging or power walking programme. This can be done easily from the yard and can be incorporated effectively into other daily routines. No special equipment is needed although investing in a pair of cushioned running trainers would be advisable, especially if you will be using hard surfaces such as Tarmac. Making use of riding school surfaces and grassy fields will also help to soften the jarring effects of jogging but extra care will be needed on uneven ground where

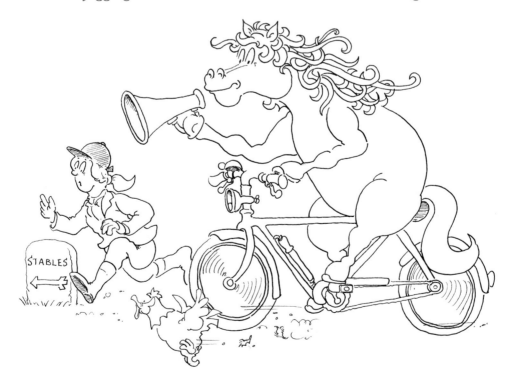

there is an increased risk of tripping and falling. The following six-week programme shows how to progress from beginner (base fitness) status through to jogging continuously for ten minutes, however, the same training principles could be applied to go further. A process known as interval training is used to gradually increase the length of each jog. Initially it can be very tempting to do more than instructed – thirty seconds may actually feel longer than you imagine! – but bear in mind that your body needs time to adapt to new stresses. Follow the programme carefully and you will progress quickly with a much reduced risk of becoming injured. Power walking – a very brisk walking action with emphasis on definite arm movements and a positive stride – can be used in place of jogging if preferred. Begin on relatively flat ground if possible and introduce hills to increase the effort as you feel ready.

Aerobic Endurance Exercises:

Note: allow twenty minutes per session to include time for warming up, cooling down and stretching.

Tips: end each jogging session with a short walk and then stretch your leg muscles while they are still warm to prevent muscle soreness.

See Chapter Ten – *Lower Body* / *Daily Stretches* – for details.

Week One:
- Walk for two minutes then jog for thirty seconds – repeat two more times
- Two or three sessions with at least one recovery day in between

Week Two:
- Walk for two minutes then jog for thirty seconds – repeat three more times
- Two or three sessions with at least one recovery day in between

Week Three:
- Walk for two minutes then jog for one minute – repeat two more times
- Three sessions with at least one recovery day in between

Week Four:
- Walk for one minute then jog for one minute – repeat four more times
- Three or four sessions

Week Five:
- Walk for thirty seconds then jog for two minutes – repeat three more times
- Three or four sessions

Week Six:
- Try jogging continuously for ten minutes. If you are using a hilly route, you might find it useful to jog on the flat and downhill sections and power walk on the uphill ones
- Three or four sessions

Tips: take a break by walking whenever needed and then continue to jog when you feel ready.

Flexibility Exercises:

The flexibility exercises introduced in Chapter Two – *Base Fitness Training* – can now be used to begin the process of improving the symmetry, or lack of it, in the rider's body. Most of us are naturally one-sided and will favour one hand over the other for everyday tasks. If you are right-handed, the chances are that you will also be right-footed, although this is not always the case. Imagine that you are about to kick a football; which foot would you use? Most of us use one side of our body far more than the other in daily activities without thinking about it and the simple process of getting dressed in the morning is a good example. You probably *always* put your stronger arm into the sleeve of a shirt or sweater first, then your stronger leg into your socks, trousers or jodhpurs first too. We become so conditioned to this pattern of movement, even just trying to dress ourselves in the opposite order to the one that comes naturally can be a surprisingly difficult challenge. Try it! If you then consider the number of daily tasks that are performed in a set way each day through this type of conditioning, it's not surprising that the problem of one-sidedness continues as we get in the saddle. If we, as riders, are unable to use both sides of our own body evenly, then how can we expect our horses to perform with symmetry and balance under us?

The flexibility exercises learned in Chapter Two – shoulder shrugs, arm circles, side stretches, hip swings, and trunk rotation – should now be repeated each time on the weaker or less favoured side of the body in order to begin addressing the imbalance. For example, if you are right-handed begin with ten shoulder shrugs using your left (weaker) arm only, follow on with ten more using your right (stronger) arm only, then repeat for another ten with your left shoulder again. Follow the same routine for all the flexibility exercises, concentrating on matching up the range of movement you have on each side of your body. You may notice differences such as being able to draw a larger or rounder circle in the air with one arm compared to the other when performing arm circles, or reaching further across in one side stretch compared to the other. By becoming aware of these problems, you are beginning the process of increasing your own body awareness. This will, in turn, improve your ability to ride with symmetry and balance as, after all, a problem can only be solved once we become aware of its existence!

It is considered correct practice to mount a horse from the left side so most riders become conditioned to this pattern of movement and find it extremely difficult to mount from the other (right) side. The tradition of mounting from the left dates back to the days of soldiers riding into battle with swords fastened to belts on their left hip as the majority were right-handed. They would mount up by placing their left foot in the stirrup in order to avoid sitting on their sword as they got into the saddle. Unless you happen to be carrying a sword as you ride, there is now no need to mount exclusively from the left! Make a habit of mounting from both sides, whether from the ground or from a mounting block, to allow your body the opportunity to work more evenly.

Another common practice is to lead your horse only from the left side. This is probably for no other reason than the majority of people being right-handed and using their stronger arm to control the horse. If you are left-handed it would make sense to lead your horse from the right side for the same reason. In my opinion, there should be no 'correct' or 'incorrect' side of the horse and every effort should be made to lead from both sides equally. However, in the interests of safety, if your horse is difficult to control from the ground then it would be wise to keep your stronger arm closest to the horse at all times. It seems an odd coincidence that the majority of horses prefer working on the left rein; could we be influencing this perhaps with our own habits?

Grooming provides another perfect opportunity to make good use of both sides of your body. When working on the right side of the horse use your right arm to groom and when working on the left side use your left arm. This is in fact correct practice but unfortunately I've witnessed many people continuing to promote their existing one-sidedness by using only their favoured arm throughout the entire grooming routine.

Great improvements in functional strength and coordination can be made by taking every opportunity to utilise both sides of your body. Many hours are spent schooling horses and training them to work evenly on both reins so it seems only fair that the same effort should be put into improving the balance across the rider's body. More time is spent off the horse than on it, so training your own muscles should not only be confined to the time actually spent in the saddle.

What's Next?

The body, whether equine or human, learns to adapt to new stresses placed upon it very quickly. If you always follow exactly the same routine, you will find that exercises which initially seemed difficult to do become relatively easy quite soon. This can be both good and bad. The good element is the fact that this adaptation allows you to advance from total beginner status to pretty competent status in only a matter of weeks in some cases but the bad element is the fact that once the adaptation has been achieved, no further progress will be made unless new stresses are introduced. This means that once you have mastered a particular exercise, a new variation or advanced version of the exercise will be needed to initiate any further improvement. The saying 'practice makes perfect' is very true but it's worth remembering that if you practise doing something badly, you will soon become very expert at doing that something badly!

Section Two of this book (Chapters Four to Nine) contains sport specific exercises to promote fitness for a range of popular equestrian sports. Many of the exercises used are relevant to more than one discipline so **Section Three** (Chapters Ten to Twelve) includes suggestions on how to put a personalised training programme together to suit your own individual needs, by choosing the exercises which will be of most benefit to you at your current level of riding. Information is also given on how to progress to the next stage of fitness and flexibility training in any riding activity by introducing a more technical approach and by including other sports to add variety and interest to your programme.

SECTION TWO

SPORT
SPECIFIC TRAINING

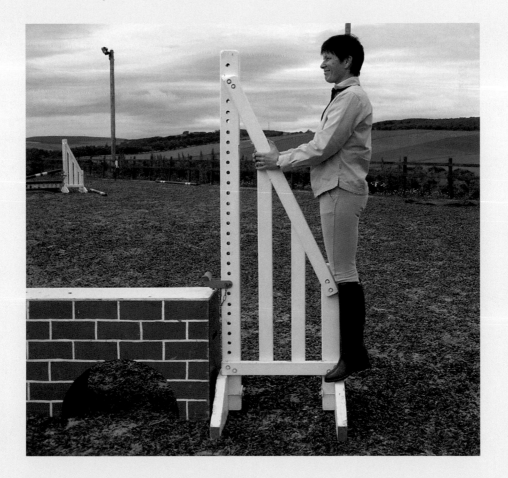

CHAPTER FOUR

RIDING SCHOOL

This chapter is aimed at the those who ride without owning their own horse. Many people ride weekly at their local riding stables, either having lessons or hacking out, and some ride only infrequently when on holiday. Riding school riders will often bemoan school horses as lethargic and 'dead to the leg' but they are, in fact, just as fit for their job as the competition horse is for his. As a novice rider gains in confidence, ability and fitness for

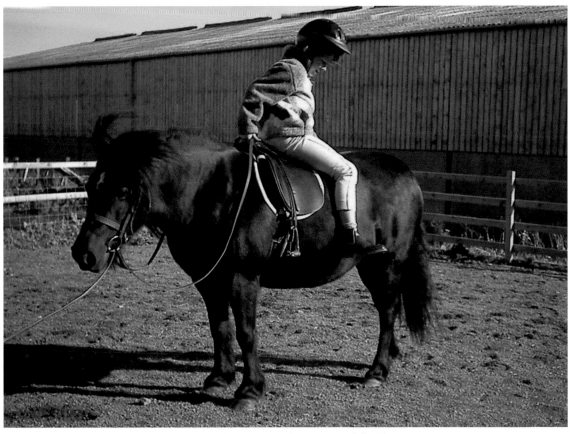

Lindsey demonstrates balance and flexibility

riding, the once 'lazy' horse will miraculously raise his game. It is my personal belief that a genuine school horse is a very clever animal indeed!

By outlining the fitness requirements of the riding school horse, it becomes easier to understand how the fitness of the rider has a direct effect on the performance of both parties. The prescribed exercises for the riding school rider are designed to promote flexibilty and strength in the areas of most concern to the new, weekly or infrequent rider so that progress can continue to be made in between rides without the need to be in the saddle.

The Horse:

Horses and ponies who work in a riding school environment will often be ridden three or four times each day and will generally only have one day off each week. They need to be fit for the job but care must be taken in training as a very fit school horse may learn to take advantage of inexperienced beginners and novice riders! The majority of their work will be in walk and trot but they must also be able to accommodate the more advanced riders who come along expecting to canter and jump in their lessons.

Unlike other equestrian disciplines, there are no general rules governing suitability for the job in terms of conformation, breed or type. Temperament is perhaps the most important consideration when choosing a horse for use in a riding school and therefore it is generally a job more suited to the older horse. This can create difficulties in terms of fitness training as many older horses will have developed lumps, bumps and old injuries through wear and tear that would often render them unsuitable for other purposes.

A gradual fittening process is needed to prepare a horse to cope with several sessions of work a day so most horses begin their training in lead-rein or beginner lessons where the pace will be slow, generally only walk, and the duration short. It takes an average of six weeks to progress from one or two slow paced half-hour sessions in a day up to three or four sessions – sometimes an hour in duration – using walk, trot and canter.

A riding school horse can be likened to a long-distance cyclist. The cyclist, just like the horse, will face many hours of repetitive movement each day. Flat sections of the cyclist's route will be relatively easy and then life will become considerably tougher when the hills appear. The horse will also face differing degrees of difficulty in each session depending on the ability of each rider. Some stages of the cyclist's journey will be more tiring than others depending on how many miles are being covered and at what point the biggest hills appear. A long hill at the end of a long day would result in a greater degree of muscle fatigue. The same would apply to a school horse if faced with an advanced jumping lesson as his fourth session of the day.

Perhaps the most difficult aspect of the work, as far as the horse is concerned, is the constant change of rider on his back. A beginner rider will not necessarily possess a sense of balance in the saddle so the horse must be able to cope with the shifting weight on board without losing his own balance. Each new rider will apply leg aids and rein aids with differing degrees of competence so it's no wonder a school horse becomes somewhat desensitised and requires a very definite signal before responding. The consequences of a riding school horse reacting instantly to every move made by a novice rider are unthinkable! Although the work may often be slow, the school horse's muscles are still being put under stress. It requires tremendous physical effort to cope with the weight of the rider moving around in the saddle and the consequent shifting of balance. If you have ever carried a wriggling child up on your shoulders, you will have some understanding of the difficulty faced by the horse. Until the new rider learns how to sit correctly and how to maintain their own balance in the saddle, the horse must work extra hard to remain balanced himself.

The process of learning how to rise to the trot inevitably results in a few sessions of bumping up and down in the saddle until the rider can feel the rhythm of the pace and learns how to move with the horse. Learning how to sit to the canter tends to involve the same process so, when you consider that a riding school horse may endure two or three hours of this each day, it should come as no surprise that back problems often occur. The more 'clockwork' the movement of the horse, the sooner the rider will learn to relax into the saddle and to feel the movement of the paces. Unfortunately, with the focus mainly on the rider at this stage of learning, the horse often goes round and round the arena in the same direction, repeating the same movements over and over again. This type of repetitive work increases the risk of overuse injuries occurring and often results in the horse becoming 'stale' as boredom sets in. Repetitive strain injuries are also common amongst long-distance cyclists so particular care is taken to build fitness and to increase mileage gradually to prevent long-term problems. By applying the same practice to the horse in training for riding school work, the risk of problems appearing is reduced greatly. Frequent changes of scenery will also allow both parties, cyclist and horse, to gain far more enjoyment from their daily journeys!

It is just as important for a school horse to warm up and prepare his muscles for work as it is for a competition horse. Warm, relaxed muscles are more pliable and therefore less susceptible to injury, plus a relaxed, flexible horse will be better equipped to cope with a less than relaxed, nervous rider. Tension in the rider's body will create a stiff, jarring, solid block in the saddle which will cause the horse to tense his own muscles, particularly in his back, to protect himself so he must be given the opportunity to warm up as freely as possible and with as little restriction as possible. This can be done by remaining in walk until the rider relaxes in the saddle. Riding slowly through a variety of school movements and changing the rein frequently will help to loosen and relax both parties but it would be of greater benefit to all concerned if the rider prepared his own muscles by warming up *before* getting into the saddle. The horse would then be spared the discomfort of an unyielding rider and the rider could get straight to work on learning new skills.

Top Training Tips from Riding School Owners:
Raise the horse's fitness level gradually by slowly increasing the hours of work and mixing the intensity of the sessions.

Keep school horses fresh by adding variety to their work and by working at more than one level e.g. include hacks as well as lessons and more experienced riders as well as beginners.

Continue to school the horses, with advanced riders, to improve and maintain flexibility and also to encourage responsiveness and discipline.

The Rider:

Most riding school riders have the opportunity to ride only once a week. Some will aspire to owning their own horse but the majority will continue to ride a variety of school horses as they continue to learn and advance their skills. Riding once a week will not be enough on its own to improve the fitness of the rider so some other form of sport specific exercise is needed between sessions to help the rider gain more from the time spent in the saddle. This will also ease the burden on the horse as a fitter, more flexible person, whether a complete beginner or an experienced rider, will be able to avoid the common riding school problem of a tired rider expecting a tired horse to carry them.

A good starting point is to follow the six-week training plan in Chapter Two – *Base Fitness Training* – with the suggested ten to fifteen minute warm-up walk around the horse's field being replaced with simply going for a walk elsewhere. On the day of your riding lesson, a warm up walk can easily be created by parking further away from the riding school and walking the last part. If we look back to the individual components of fitness introduced in Chapter One, we can then ascertain which areas are of particular importance to the riding school rider.

Aerobic Endurance:
Many people find that they get quite out of breath when first learning to ride. This could be due to a lack of fitness in general or the fact that your body will always be working much harder when learning something new compared to something familiar. Even Kelly Holmes would find herself as puffed as the next person if she'd never ridden before! Feeling out of breath will undoubtedly get in the way of progress so improving cardiovascular fitness will be of benefit to the rider.

Anaerobic / Muscular Endurance:
Not an essential component of fitness for the riding school rider.

Strength:
As with all riding, pure strength is not necessary at any level. In some cases, new riders will use strength to grip the saddle, in place of using balance, through fear of falling off. The consequent tension in the rider's body will prevent them from relaxing and will soon tire them out. Core strength, and stability in the back and stomach muscles, is important to allow the rider to maintain good posture and a correct position in the saddle. However, flexibility must also be maintained, along with core strength, to prevent a rigid, unyielding posture forming which would limit the rider's movement.

Speed:
The rider has no need to develop speed in his own muscles when riding.

Power:
No need for power when riding.

Body Composition:
Excess body fat creates general health concerns but need not prevent someone from learning to ride. A heavier rider requires a heavier or stronger horse to carry them so the choice of available mount at your local riding school may become limited if you become an overweight rider. Body fat around the joints also restricts mobility and will make it more difficult to move with the horse or to apply effective aids. By improving body composition, the rider will feel more comfortable in the saddle and, by becoming healthier in general, they are likely to gain far more from their riding.

Flexibility:
An absolutely essential component of fitness for all riders. As the new rider becomes more flexible, they will develop a greater feel for the movement of the horse and will learn to relax into the saddle. Riding school horses are

notoriously stiff due to the nature of their work but, as outlined above, this can often be the result of a stiff, unyielding rider. A more flexible rider becomes a more effective rider and will be able to help the horse in turn.

Riding School Rider Exercises:

The following exercises are designed for those who ride just once a week or infrequently. It is necessary to continue training the muscle groups used in riding, even when not in the saddle, so that progress can continue to be made from one session to the next. Most weekly riders will experience aches and pains after a lesson and unfortunately the same aches tend to hang around for a day or two each time. By training the same riding muscles in-between sessions, they will quickly become better conditioned to cope with the next ride and the aches will soon become a thing of the past. The following joint mobility exercises, along with the flexibility exercises introduced in Chapter Two – *Base Fitness Training,* provide an ideal warm-up to prepare your body for riding before getting into the saddle at the start of each ride and also between lessons.

Joint Mobility Exercises:

Your body must always be warm before exercising. These joint mobility exercises will help to warm up the muscles and loosen the joints in preparation for riding but can also be used to improve mobility in general. Start slowly and take care not to overdo any movement.

> **Tips:** try to spend a few minutes working through the following routine on a daily basis.

Neck:
- Gently tilt your head forwards to position your chin on your chest – this will stretch the muscles at the back of your neck
- Return to the start position and then turn your head to look to the right – this will stretch the muscles on the left side of your neck
- Return to the start position and then turn your head to look to the left – this will stretch the muscles on the right side of your neck
- Keep good posture, take your time, stay relaxed and breathe normally.

Elbows:
- Gently swing your right hand towards your right shoulder and then return to the start position
- Gently swing your left hand towards your left shoulder and then return to the start position

- Continue to swing alternate arms several more times to loosen up the elbow joints

Wrists:
- Gently rotate your right wrist through its full range of motion
- Gently rotate your left wrist through its full range of motion
- Repeat several rotations in both a clockwise and anti-clockwise direction to loosen the wrist joints – you may notice your stronger arm wrist appears to be naturally more mobile so work on matching things up

Trunk / Spine:
- Stand with your feet placed hip-width apart and keep a slight bend in your knees
- Place your hands on your hips and rotate through your waist to look around to the right
- Return to face the front and then rotate to look around to the left
- Repeat several times to stretch the muscles of the trunk and loosen the joints in the spine
- Keep good posture, take your time, stay relaxed and breathe normally

Hips / Pelvis:
- Stand with your feet placed hip-width apart and keep a slight bend in your knees
- Place your hands on your hips and gently move your hips in a circular motion as if exercising with a hula-hoop!
- Repeat several times rotating in both a clockwise and anti-clockwise direction
- Keep good posture, take your time, stay relaxed and breathe normally

Knees:
- Lean on something for balance and then stand on one leg – keep a slight bend in the knee of the standing leg
- Gently swing the other leg by raising your heel towards your bottom and then relaxing down again
- Repeat several times to loosen the knee joint and then change position to repeat using the other leg
- Keep good posture, take your time, stay relaxed and breathe normally

Ankles:
- Lean against something for balance or sit down
- Gently rotate your right ankle through its full range of movement
- Repeat with the left ankle

• Repeat several times in both a clockwise and anti-clockwise direction to loosen the ankle joints – as with the wrists, you may notice your stronger leg ankle appears to be naturally more mobile so try to match things up

Core Stability / Strengthening Exercises:
Follow the above joint mobility exercises with the flexibility exercises learned in Chapter Two – shoulder shrugs / arm circles / side stretches / hip swings / and trunk rotation – and then add the following strengthening exercises.

> **Tips:** aim to exercise two or three times a week between riding lessons.

> **Note:** a guide to the location and function of the muscles can be found at the end of Chapter One.

A Leg at Each Corner: (*see* pictures 6a and 6b)
This exercise may take some practise as you will probably feel quite unstable on your first attempt. The core muscles – abdominals, obliques and lower back – will work hard to stabilise you even while you practise so you will still continue to strengthen your body's core.
• Position yourself on the floor as in the picture

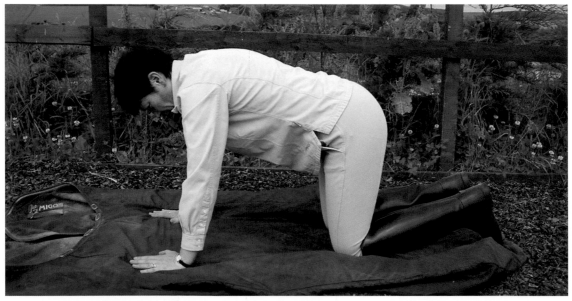

6a A leg at each corner

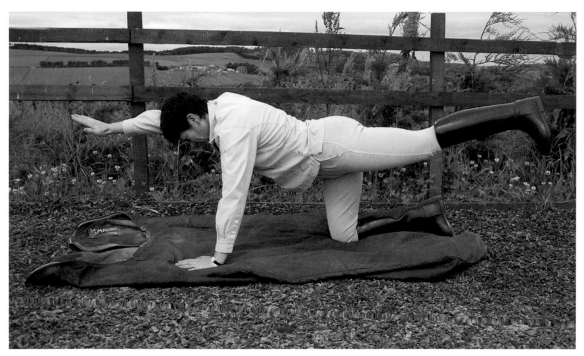

6b Raise opposite arm and leg simultaneously

- Keep your head, neck and spine in line by keeping good posture in your back and looking towards the floor (raising your head will cause your back to sag)
- Raise opposite arm and leg (e.g. right arm and left leg) simultaneously and straighten each limb as much as possible to form a straight line with your back
- Hold for ten seconds, stay relaxed and breathe normally
- Return to the start position and repeat using the other arm and leg
- Repeat the whole exercise once more

Bucking Bronco: (*see* pictures 7a and 7b overleaf)
This exercise conditions the core muscles, particularly abdominals, and increases mobility in the spine.

- Position yourself on the floor as in the picture
- Tuck your chin in towards your chest
- Take a deep breath in through your nose and arch your back as you pull in your stomach muscles towards your spine – hold for a few seconds
- Breathe out through your mouth as you allow your back to relax back down
- Keep your head, neck and spine in line (avoid sagging) but continue to hold in your stomach muscles towards your spine as you breathe out
- Repeat twice more – remember to breathe

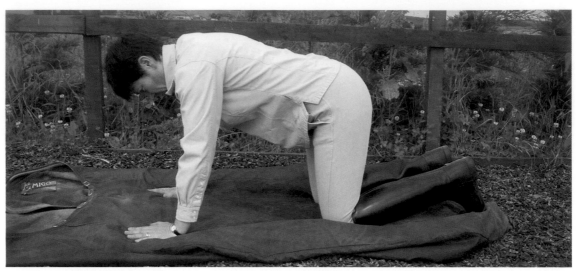

7a Bucking bronco

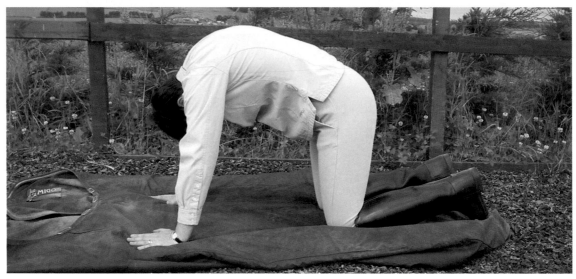

7b Arch your back as you pull in your stomach muscles

Fat Horse Squats: (*see* pictures 8a and 8b)
This exercise strengthens the leg muscles – quadriceps, hamstrings, gluteals, calves – and increases the flexibility of the adductor muscles.

> **Tips:** in place of a lunge whip, use any item strong enough to aid balance e.g. broom, chair back, door frame.

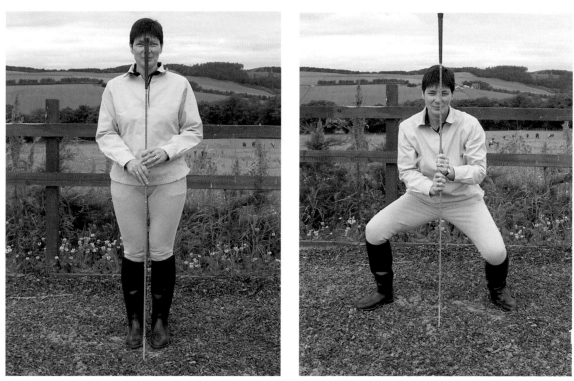

8a Fat horse squats　　　　　*8b Step to the side to squat down*

• Start with your feet together and then step out to the side with one foot, allowing your toe to turn out slightly
• Squat down as low as you comfortably can to feel a stretch on the inner thigh muscles
• Keep an upright posture (straight back) as you squat and breathe out through your mouth as you hold the stretch for a few seconds
• Breathe in through your nose as you return to the start position – feet together – then repeat the exercise by stepping out to the other side using the other foot
• Repeat the whole exercise twice more and try to step out a little wider or squat a little lower each time to increase the workload

Heels Down: (*see* pictures 9a, 9b and 9c overleaf)
This exercise isolates the calf muscles and will help to develop greater strength and flexibility, making it easier to ride with the heel lower than the toe in the stirrup.

Tips: in place of a jump wing, use a step or something similar to stand on instead.

- Stand with your toes on the edge of a jump wing (or step) as in the picture – lean on something for balance
- Keep your legs straight (knees locked) and raise your heels to go up on to your toes
- Allow your heels to drop towards the floor until you feel a stretch in your calf muscles – hold for ten seconds
- Repeat the whole exercise twice more
- Keep good posture, take your time, stay relaxed and breathe normally

The above exercises could easily be done indoors in the comfort of your own home and between riding lessons but, to further enhance your actual riding time, make it a routine practice to warm up your body immediately before each riding lesson – be aware that cold muscles are less flexible than warm muscles. The process of warming your horse up is unlikely to warm up your own body effectively, especially in cold weather, so spending a few minutes just getting yourself on the move and mobilising your joints with a few exercises will ensure that you are ready for action as soon as you get into the saddle. Remember that your horse will also appreciate the feeling of a relaxed, supple rider on his back, rather than a stiff, unyielding one.

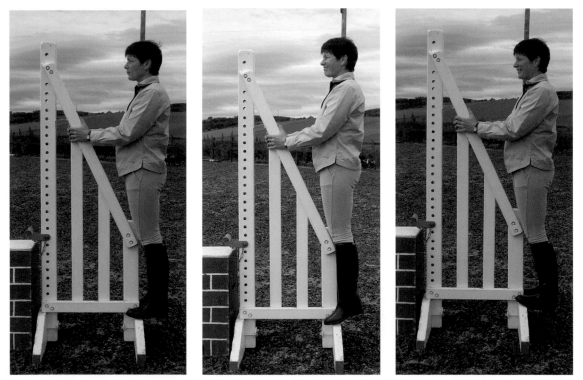

9a Position toes on the edge of a step

9b Raise your heels to work the calves

9c Lower your heels to stretch the calves

Case Study:

Rider – Kimberley Carter
Age – 31 years

Riding Experience:

Kimberley rode as a child from age six to ten years and then stopped when she lost confidence after a fall. After a break of twenty years she decided to take riding lessons again when her own six-year-old daughter expressed an interest. Having not participated in any form of exercise for several years, Kimberley discovered that each riding lesson was leaving her feeling stiff and sore for several days in muscles she'd forgotten she had. The following programme was devised to help condition the muscles and to alleviate the aches by preparing carefully before each ride and then continuing to develop appropriate postural strength and flexibility in-between lessons.

Saturday:
One hour group riding lesson.

1. Ten minutes before the lesson:
Joint mobility exercises – neck, elbows, wrists, trunk / spine, hips / pelvis, knees and ankles (as detailed in rider exercises).
Flexibility exercises – shoulder shrugs, arm circles, side stretches, hip swings and trunk rotation (Chapter Two).
2. Within ten minutes after the lesson:
Daily stretches – upper body and lower body (Chapter Ten).

Sunday:
1. Family walk of twenty to thirty minutes.
2. Daily stretches – upper body and lower body (Chapter Ten).

Monday:
1. Walk / housework / gardening / at least ten minutes of warm-up activity.
2. All joint mobility exercises, flexibility exercises, and daily stretches as Saturday.

Tuesday:
Rest day.

Wednesday:
1.   Walk / housework / gardening / at least ten minutes of warm-up activity.
2. Core stability / strengthening exercises – a leg at each corner, bucking bronco, fat horse squats and heels down (as detailed in rider exercises).
3. Daily stretches – upper body and lower body (Chapter Ten).

Thursday:
1. Brisk walk or at least ten minutes of warming up activity.
2. All advanced stretches – lying hamstring, adductor, lower back and gluteal, and hip flexor muscles (Chapter Ten).

Friday:
1. One hour swimming session with the children.
2. All daily stretches – upper body and lower body (Chapter Ten).

Summary of Fitness Training for Riding School Riders:

• Aim to exercise the riding muscles regularly between lessons / rides
• Warm up your own body before getting into the saddle each time
• Get into a regular routine of joint mobility and stretching exercises to improve and maintain flexibility for riding and to minimise aches and pains
• Train to improve cardiovascular and general fitness to avoid fatigue
• Train to increase strength in the core muscles and to improve flexibility as this will promote a relaxed, balanced and secure position in the saddle

CHAPTER FIVE

DRESSAGE

When asked to think of a dressage horse, most people conjure up an image of a highly trained horse and rider combination competing in top hat and tails at Olympic level. However, dressage is an important part of basic training for *all* horses in *all* disciplines at *all* levels and is simply known as flatwork training. Work on the flat teaches the horse how to balance himself; how to move forwards freely; how to remain balanced through turns and changes of pace; and it also helps to develop muscular strength, flexibility and coordination. These lessons are of equal importance to the

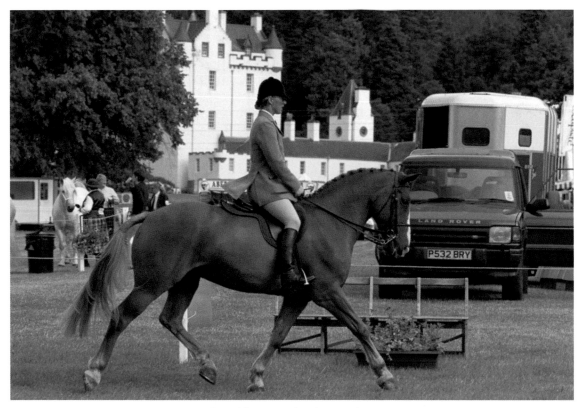

A relaxed horse and rider combination

dressage rider! All the above skills form the basic foundations of any training programme and flatwork – or dressage – movements allow the horse to continue progressing through his working life by remaining supple, relaxed, responsive and obedient.

The Horse:

To be able to compete at Preliminary Standard in British Dressage tests a horse must be a minimum of four years old. Most horses (and riders) will begin at this level and then work progressively through the advancing levels as their abilities increase. On average, horses competing at Advanced Standard will be over eight years old so at least four years of specific training are necessary to enable a horse to perform at this level. In all competitions the horse will be judged on :

1. Paces – freedom and regularity.
2. Impulsion – elasticity of the steps; desire to move forwards; and the suppleness of the back.
3. Submission – acceptance of the aids; confidence; balance; and lightness and ease of the movements.

Clearly, to perform well in dressage the horse must score well in all three categories so his training must encompass all areas. A degree of potential ability will be dictated by conformation and certain breeds are favoured over others for their natural characteristics. The warmblood breeds often feature at top level for this reason but it may well be due to their temperament as much as their physical attributes. In theory, any horse with good basic conformation and a straight action should be able to perform well in the dressage arena when given the appropriate training. The difference between an adequate performance and a winning performance could well be more to do with mental attitude than physical ability. This should be remembered when planning a training programme for a dressage horse as hour upon hour of intensive schooling work within the same arena will probably not inspire much enjoyment. Horses, just like people, learn best when all their senses are stimulated and they actually enjoy the process of learning.

Dressage is often referred to as equine ballet so you could liken the dressage horse to a ballet dancer. Dancers, just like the dressage horse, require both muscular strength and immense flexibility to be able to perform at top level. They will go through hours of intensive training on a daily basis but the most important element of every routine is the warm-up. Muscles must be thoroughly warm and relaxed before they are asked to work hard as failure to prepare the body for the stresses of exercise will generally result in injury. Warming up has to be a gradual process so it takes time but it's not unusual to see riders walking once around the edge of the arena and then expecting their horse to instantly begin working on canter pirouettes! Depending on the individual, it could easily take twenty minutes or more of gentle working in to truly warm up the horse's muscles from the inside out. The muscles also need to be relaxed to work efficiently so asking for too much too soon will certainly prevent this from happening. A tense horse, particularly if tense through their back muscles, will achieve little in their schooling session and may even become injured. So, even if you are pushed for time, it is a far better plan to spend twenty minutes warming up slowly to then experience ten minutes of good quality work rather than to spend thirty minutes rushing around to achieve absolutely nothing but frustration and disappointment. During periods of intense schooling, the muscles are put under great stress so they will need to be given the opportunity throughout a training session to stretch and relax from time to time to prevent tension. Think how good it feels to stretch your own muscles after an exercise session or even how much of a relief it is to stretch after being stuck in one position for a long time.

A horse training and competing at Preliminary Standard should be able to demonstrate working paces in walk, trot and canter. At Novice Standard medium paces are introduced, at Elementary Standard collected paces are required, and extended paces appear at Medium Standard. Without the ability to remain balanced, light on the forehand, working from the hindquarters, supple in the back muscles and relaxed, the horse will not be able to carry himself, let alone the rider, in even the working paces. Without the working paces, the medium paces can't develop and so on all the way through the levels. It is therefore absolutely essential to train the horse progressively so as to allow time for the muscles to develop accordingly. The skills developed at each stage along the way are the necessary building blocks to allow the horse to improve and without those strong foundations the whole structure will collapse sooner or later.

At Preliminary Standard school movements are simple. Transitions are progressive (walk to trot then trot to canter etc.) and often performed between markers to prevent rushing. The degree of difficulty involved in the movements increases as the horse progresses through the levels so greater degrees of fitness and flexibility are also needed. Changes of pace are expected to be more precise, often on the marker, and direct transitions (walk to canter etc.) are required. Again, without the ability to bend evenly in both directions or the balance and co-ordination to perform accurately at Preliminary Standard, the building blocks are not in place to allow progression and cracks will appear in the structure at some stage.

It becomes quite obvious that years of skilled preparation must go into the training of a competitive dressage horse. The British Dressage system of tests provides a useful means of progressing sensibly from one level to the next by introducing new skills at appropriate stages in the horse's training. The same system can be used by all riders with an interest in schooling their horse whether they intend to compete or not.

Top Training Tips from Dressage Riders:
Achieve perfection in the basics before introducing any other movements.

Allow the horse time to mature mentally as well as physically.

Use variety in training to add interest and enjoyment e.g. working outdoors on hills can help develop muscle tone and balance; working over ground poles can encourage elevation and lengthening of paces; negotiating natural obstacles such as rough ground, puddles, gateways etc. can aid learning in lateral work.

The Rider:

No matter how well trained or schooled the horse, the ability to move freely with balance will be lost if the rider sits in such a way as to obstruct the natural movement of the horse's muscles. Tension in the rider's body, 'fixed' hands, crooked seat position, one-sided use of aids – the list could go on and on – will all influence the horse's way of going and make applying appropriate signals or aids virtually impossible. A score is also given to the rider when taking part in dressage competitions at any level and the judge will award points on the rider's position and seat along with the correct application and effectiveness of the aids. When you consider the long list of criteria the horse will be judged on, the rider appears to get off quite lightly. However, without a supple and effective rider the horse is unlikely to perform at his best so both parties must work together in harmony to achieve the desired results.

The importance of warming up the horse's muscles before asking them to work has already been stressed so the same emphasis must now be placed upon the warming up of the rider's own muscles. The time spent in the saddle whilst warming up the horse is not an effective means of warming up the rider. Any movement that gradually increases the body's core temperature and slowly increases the heart and breathing rate for at least five minutes, preferably ten, will suffice. The joint mobility exercises detailed in Chapter Four can be used as a useful warm up or see Chapter Ten – *Warm Up Routines for Riders* – for further suggestions.

By referring back to the list of fitness components in Chapter One, we can now ascertain which elements are of specific relevance to the dressage rider and devise suitable exercises to develop the appropriate skills to help maximise performance.

Aerobic Endurance:

A dressage test may last anything from four minutes up to around seven minutes so it cannot be classed as an endurance event. However, I've witnessed many riders collapse into breathless heaps on the floor at the end of a test so clearly a degree of cardiovascular fitness is needed to prevent this. In some cases the breathlessness is a result of tension or even breath-holding but with far reaching consequences for the rider and also the horse.

Anaerobic / Muscular Endurance:

As there are no movements involved in dressage riding that require speed or repeated use of a particular group of muscles, anaerobic endurance is not a vital component.

Strength:

Pure strength is not a necessary requirement for riding. In fact, the use of strength could be considered detrimental to performance if used as a means of applying force. To be able to maintain a good position in the saddle, or a 'deep seat', the rider must develop a strong core which involves recruiting the muscles which form the trunk of the body, mainly abdominal and back. However, to be effective, the core muscles must also remain flexible otherwise the rider becomes 'fixed' and immobile.

Speed:

This is not an essential component of fitness for any rider.

Power:

Unlike the horse, a dressage rider has no need to develop power in any muscle group.

Body Composition:

Excessive body fat will affect the rider's general fitness due to the associated health implications. It will also affect the rider's ability to sit close and to move freely with the horse as the fat stored under the skin may limit the range of movement available around the joints.

Flexibility:

A vital fitness component for the dressage rider. Flexibility allows the rider to develop a greater 'feel' in the saddle; the ability to move with the horse; and a more sympathetic use of seat and leg aids.

Dressage Rider Exercises:

The following exercises are designed to improve the most important elements of fitness for dressage riding – joint mobility, flexibility and core strength. Practise the exercises by incorporating the movements into your aerobic endurance training routine (base fitness training) so that you can remain on the move and keep your muscles warm. Alternatively, after warming up, aim to perform each exercise for just enough time to feel the targeted muscle group working (generally between ten and twenty repetitions) or try the *Dressage Drills* detailed later in this chapter. Remember the idea is to promote movement, increase flexibility and improve fitness for riding – not to wear you out!

> **Note:** a guide to the location and function of the muscles can be found at the end of Chapter One.

Body Stretch – to remove tension from the whole body (*see* pictures 10a and 10b)

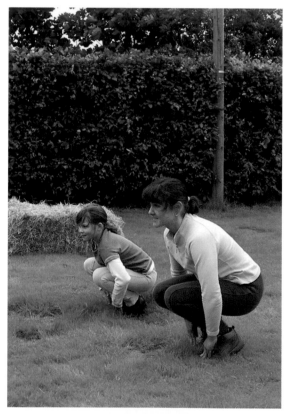

10a Body stretch

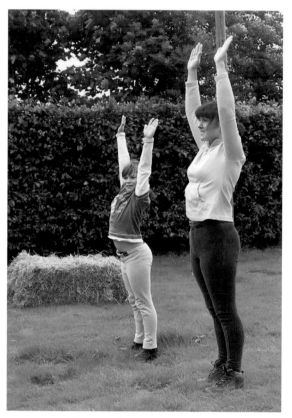

10b Breathe in as you stretch

- Stand with your feet together
- Bend your knees to reach down and touch your toes
- Straighten up as you stretch your whole body by reaching towards the sky – take a deep breath in through your nose as you stretch up
- Breathe out through your mouth as you relax back to the starting position

Heel Kicks – to mobilise the knee joints and work the hamstring muscles (*see* pictures 11a and 11b)

- Walk forwards using normal stride length
- Kick alternate heels up towards your bottom as you walk along
- Keep good posture and breathe normally

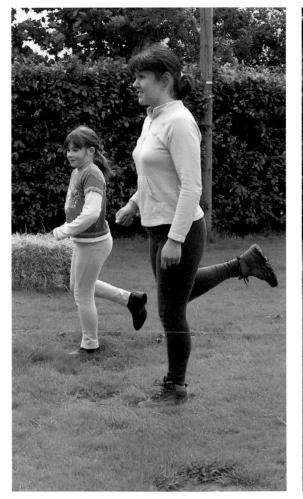

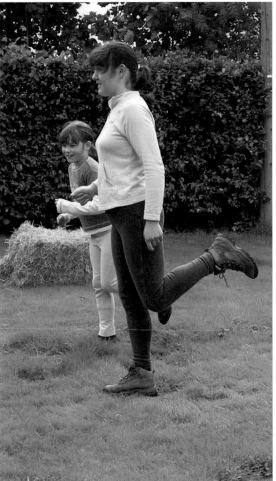

11a Heel kicks   *11b Kick alternate heels as you walk*

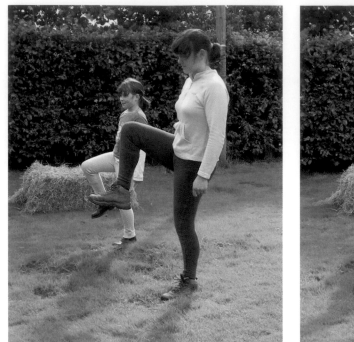

| 12a Knee lifts | 12b Lift alternate knees as you walk |

Knee Lifts – to mobilise the hip joints
and work the hip flexor and quadricep muscles (*see* pictures 12a and 12b)

- Walk forwards using normal stride length
- Lift alternate knees up towards your chest (or as high as possible) as you walk along
- Keep good posture and breathe normally

Travelling Wide Squats – to work the leg muscles – hamstrings, quadriceps, gluteals, calves – and to stretch the adductor muscles (*see* pictures 13a and 13b)

- Travelling sideways – take a step to the side (right or left leg leading the way)
- Squat down, sticking your bottom out behind you as if aiming to sit on a chair
- Stand up and bring your feet together to then take another step and repeat – this keeps you travelling
- The wider your step and/or the lower your squat, the more intense the stretch becomes
- Breathe out through your mouth as you squat down and in through your nose as you stand up each time

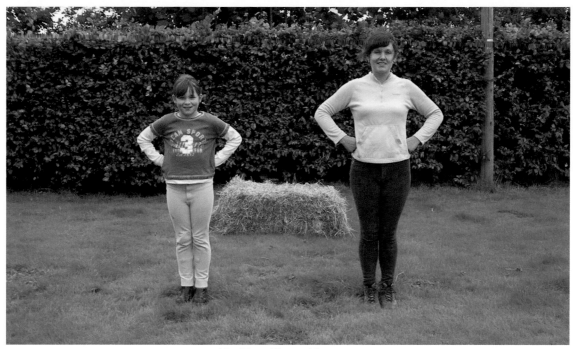

13a Travelling wide squats

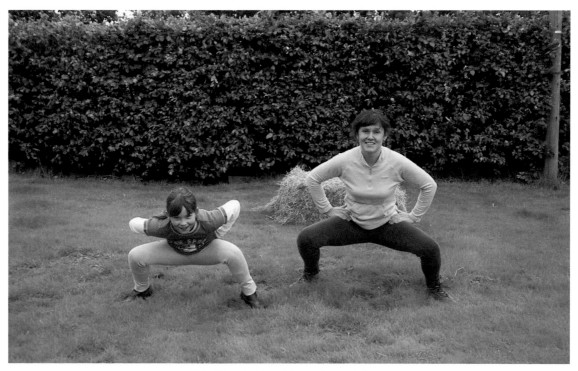

13b Step to the side and squat down

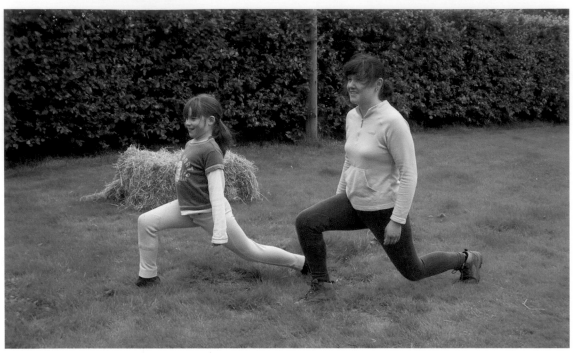

14a Travelling front lunge right

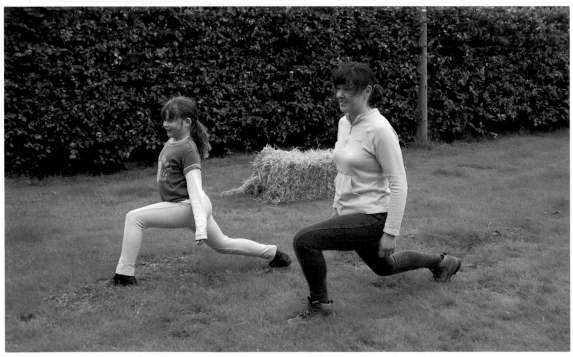

14b Travelling front lunge left

Travelling Front Lunges – to work the leg muscles – quadriceps, calves –and to stretch the hip flexor muscles (*see* pictures 14a and 14b)

- Travelling forwards – take a big step with either leg in front of you
- Hold this position and gently lower the knee of the back leg towards the ground
- Both knees should be bent and allow the heel of the back foot to lift from the ground
- A stretch should be felt at the top of the thigh on the back leg - hold for ten seconds
- Stand up and continue forwards by taking a big step with the other leg to repeat the exercise
- The bigger your step, the more intense the stretch becomes
- Keep an upright posture in your upper body and breathe out through your mouth as you stretch and in through your nose as you stand up each time

The Plank – to strengthen the core – abdominal and back – muscles (*see* picture 15)

- Position yourself on the bale with elbows under shoulders for balance
- Turn your body into a plank by keeping your head and neck in line with your spine and keeping just your toes on the ground
- Hold your stomach muscles in towards your spine but continue to breathe normally
- Hold this position for one minute if possible – rest by placing your knees on the ground whenever necessary

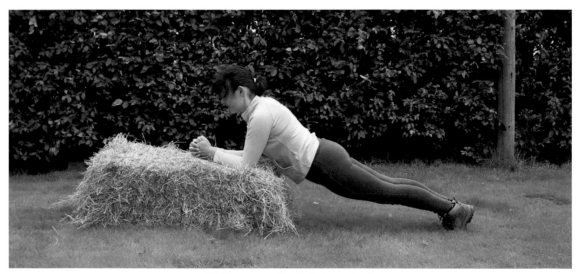

15 Turn your body into a plank

Dressage Drills:

To make your exercise sessions more fun, try turning your riding arena into your very own personal gym by putting yourself through your paces on your own two feet with the following *Dressage Drills* for preliminary, novice, elementary and advanced exercisers! Each drill contains a combination of the above exercises and those already learned in Chapter Two – *Base Fitness Training* – so experiment with each level and progress at your own pace. All you need is a set of dressage markers in your school or in the field – the bigger the school, the harder you'll work. Why not get some friends together and do a group drill to music?

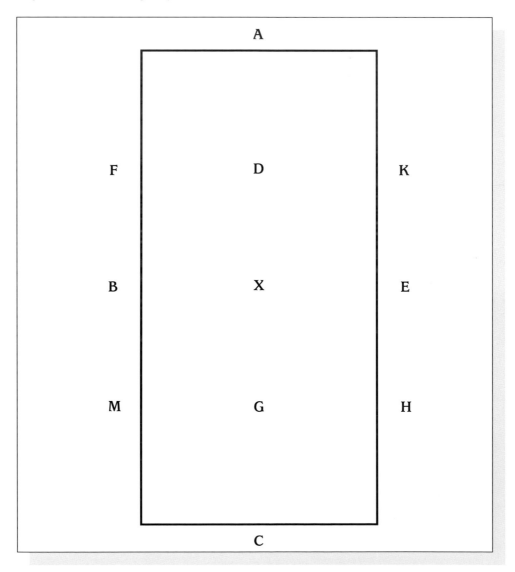

Preliminary Drill One

A	Enter at brisk walk
X	Halt, whole body stretch
C	Track left – brisk walk
A	Circle left 20 metres (65 feet) diameter
F to B	Arm circles right
B to M	Arm circles left
HXF	Lengthened strides in brisk walk
K to E	Alternate leg heel kicks
E to H	Alternate leg knee lifts
C	Circle right 20 metres (65 feet) diameter
MXK	Lengthened strides in brisk walk
A	Side stretches – to right x 5 / to left x 5
AFB	Brisk walk
B	Left leg hip swings x 5
B to X	Half 10 metre (32 feet) circle left
X to E	Half 10 metre (32 feet) circle right
E	Right leg hip swings x 5
EHCM	Brisk walk
M to B	Travelling wide squats – left leg leading
B to F	Travelling wide squats – right leg leading
F	Skip
A	Skip down centre line
X	Halt, whole body stretch

Novice Drill Two

A	Enter at brisk walk
X	Halt, whole body stretch
C	Track left – brisk walk
HEK	Arm circles – alternate arms (backstroke)
A	Down centre line – brisk walk
C	Track right
MBF	Arm circles – alternate arms
A	Side stretches – to right x 5 / to left x 5
A	Circle right 20 metres (65 feet) diameter – easy jog
KXM	Lengthened strides in brisk walk

Novice Drill Two (continued)

C	Hip swings – right leg x 5 / left leg x 5
C	Circle left 20 metres (65 feet) diameter – easy jog
H to X	Alternate leg heel kicks – brisk walk
X to F	Alternate leg knee lifts – brisk walk
A	Down centre line
D to X	Travelling wide squats right
X to G	Travelling wide squats left
G	Halt, whole body stretch

Elementary Drill Three
(a bale is needed at A in this drill)

A	Enter at brisk walk or jog
X	Halt, whole body stretch
C	Track left – brisk walk or jog
HEK	Brisk walk or jog
A to X	Half 20 metre (65 feet) circle left – arm circles right
X to C	Half 20 metre (65 feet) circle right – arm circles left
MBF	Brisk walk or jog
A	Side stretches – to right x 10 / to left x 10
K to E	Travelling wide squats left
E	Circle right 10 metres (32 feet) diameter – easy jog
E to H	Travelling wide squats right
C	Hip swings – right leg x 10 / left leg x 10
M to X	Alternate leg heel kicks in jog
X to K	Alternate leg knee lifts in walk or jog
A	The plank
F to B	Skip
B	Circle left 10 metres (32 feet) diameter – easy jog
B to M	Skip
MCH	Brisk walk
HXF	Lengthened strides in brisk walk or jog
A	Down centre line – walk or jog
X to G	Travelling front lunges
G	Halt, whole body stretch

Advanced Drill Four

(a bale and a lunge whip are needed at A for this drill)

A	Enter at jog
X	Halt, whole body stretch
C	Track right – easy jog
MXK	Easy Jog
A	Down centre line
D to X	Walk – arm circles right
X to G	Walk – arm circles left
C	Track left – easy jog
HXF	Easy jog
A	Side stretches – to right x 10 / to left x 10
AK	Easy jog
KEH	Alternate leg heel kicks in jog
C	Hip swings – right leg x 10 / left leg x 10
CM	Easy jog
M to B	Alternate leg knee lifts in jog
B to K	Easy jog
A	Trunk rotation – to right x 5 / to left x 5
A	Three looped serpentine – skip or jog
CHB	Travelling front lunges
BFA	Easy jog
A to X	Travelling wide squats left
X to A	Travelling wide squats right
A	The plank
A	Skip down centre line
G	Halt, whole body stretch

Aim to exercise at least two or three times each week. By using a combination of the above exercises along with the routines learned in Chapters Two and Three it is possible to create your own programme of exercises to suit your own particular circumstances. Mix and match the contents of each programme to make use of the elements that will be of most benefit to you at your current level of fitness – Chapter Twelve contains suggestions on personalising your programme. Your body adapts quickly to new stresses placed upon it so aim to use a variety of exercises to promote further progress and also to keep things interesting. Remember that as little as ten minutes of activity on a regular basis will go a long way towards improving your fitness for dressage.

Case Study:

Rider – Karen Shimmins
Age – 23

Riding Experience:

Karen has ridden once or twice a week at her local riding school since childhood and has recently bought her own horse. Karen's aim is to compete in affiliated dressage competitions and the following programme was designed to improve her fitness for riding as she found the transition from riding a couple of times a week to riding five or six times a week quite difficult. Her new horse has already competed at Preliminary Standard and Karen wants to make sure that her own stiffness does not interfere with her horse's natural paces.

Saturday:

One hour riding lesson on own horse.

1. Ten minutes before lesson:
(When warm) all flexibility exercises detailed in Chapter Two – shoulder shrugs, arm circles, side stretches, hip swings and trunk rotation.
2. Within ten minutes after lesson:
All daily stretches – upper body and lower body (Chapter Ten).

Sunday:

1. Ride as normal.
2. *Dressage Drill* – Preliminary Drill One.
3. All daily stretches – upper body and lower body (Chapter Ten).

Monday:

1. No riding.
2. After a soak in the bath – all advanced stretches – lying hamstring, adductors, lower back and gluteals, and hip flexors (Chapter Ten).

Tuesday:

1. Ride as normal.
2. *Dressage Drill* – Novice Drill Two.
3. All daily stretches – upper body and lower body (Chapter Ten).

Wednesday:
1. Before ride:
Brisk walk / grooming etc. – at least ten minutes of warming up activity.
All flexibility exercises as Saturday.
2. During ride: (hack out if time permits after work).
Dismount and lead on foot for five minutes at least once on route.
3. After ride:
All daily stretches – upper body and lower body (Chapter Ten).

Thursday:
1. Ride as normal.
2. *Dressage Drill* – Elementary Drill Three.
3. All daily stretches – upper body and lower body (Chapter Ten).

Friday:
As Monday.

Summary of Rider Fitness Training for Dressage:

- Train for aerobic endurance, core strength and flexibility
- Get into a regular stretching routine to increase body awareness
- Train both sides of your body to improve balance, symmetry, and effectiveness in the saddle
- Train to be able to maintain good posture and a relaxed position in the saddle – be aware of the detrimental effects of tension in the rider's body
- Warm up your own body before getting into the saddle

CHAPTER SIX

SHOW JUMPING

Horses are natural jumpers in that they have the physical ability to leap over obstacles but fortunately for us they generally choose not to use this ability unless influenced by a rider – otherwise how would we keep them in fields?

Young riders will often compare their abilities by asking, 'How high can you jump?' and the rider who has jumped the highest fence is generally considered to be the most skilled. Obviously, this is not a good method of judging a rider's ability! The horse is the athlete who must actually jump the fence, not the rider, so his level of fitness will have a direct effect on performance and ability but the influence of the rider cannot be ignored. Both horse and rider must train specifically for their sport and both parties must be equally fit and flexible to create a winning combination.

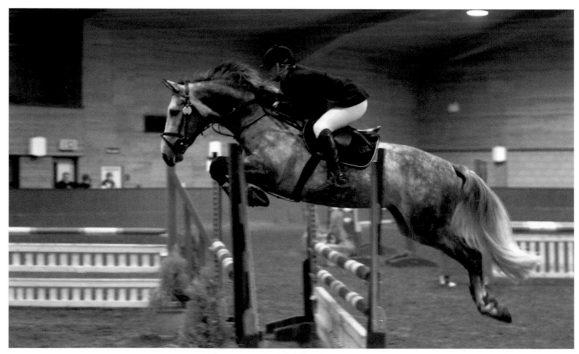

A fit and flexible combination

The Horse:

A horse must be a minimum of four years old to compete under British Show Jumping Association (BSJA) rules and classes for this age group are designed to promote confidence and develop skills without over-taxing the young horse's body. A huge variety of classes are then offered at affiliated competitions but in general, the height and width of the fences will increase as the horse progresses.

The horse's general conformation will dictate potential jumping ability but good basic conformation will also limit the risk of injuries occurring in training and competition. To negotiate a course of fences successfully, the horse must have the necessary strength to take off; the flexibility to bascule over the fence; the balance to maintain a rhythm between fences; and a combination of all three to cope with the tremendous stress placed upon the body, particularly the forelimbs, when landing after a fence. To achieve this, an appropriate and progressive training programme must be in place to ensure the horse is conditioned carefully in preparation for the rigours of the sport at each level.

A show jumping horse could be likened to a human 400 metre hurdler. Both need significant physical ability to negotiate obstacles but they also need to be skilled in pace control and stride judgement in order to cover the ground at optimum speed, yet still maintain the essential coordination necessary to provide accurate take-offs and to ensure efficient clearance each time. The fitness training programme in both cases begins with strengthening, conditioning and flexibility exercises on the flat.

Flatwork training ensures that the young horse develops the necessary skills to allow him to maintain balance in all paces and through transitions, including variations – lengthening and shortening – within a pace. He may have natural ability and a bold jump but if he is unable to control his movements between fences he is unlikely to progress far before mistakes will be made and a lack of confidence will then creep in. The successful show jumping horse requires just as much strength as the dressage horse so an appropriate period of time must be allowed in the training programme to develop this. Skills on the flat should be mastered before jumping training takes over. The more ability the horse has on the flat, in terms of working from his hind quarters and collecting his paces, the more his jumping ability is likely to improve. Greater flexibility will also allow for more scope when jumping; allow tighter turns to be negotiated without losing balance; and limit the risk of injuries occurring.

Many talented horses unfortunately suffer the consequences of being 'over faced' in the early stages of their jumping career. This can also be the case for many human athletes and could be avoided by remembering the old saying, 'Don't run before you can walk.' Both parties, human and equine, must gain confidence in their abilities over simple courses and lower obstacles before being asked to do more. Sufficient training time must be allowed to develop physical skills progressively and also to allow the athlete to become mentally prepared for the rigours of their sport. It doesn't take long for a human hurdler to begin backing off the hurdles if they have experienced a few problems such as misjudging the take-off point and hitting the hurdle or, even worse, falling over the hurdle. It is exactly the same for a horse who experiences a few hard knocks or even a fall – confidence is lost. The rider has a large part to play in avoiding this situation by planning an appropriate training programme and also by making sure that they sit correctly in the saddle when asking their horse to jump. If the rider constantly thumps down on the horse's back after each fence or yanks hard on the horse's mouth through being left behind the movement over each fence, it won't take long before the horse begins to associate jumping with pain – can you blame the horse for then refusing?

Top Training Tips from Show Jumping Riders:
Train all horses in dressage before introducing jumps – basic flatwork skills must be mastered before progressing to jumping as they will be required to link the fences!

Use variety in training to condition the horse's muscles e.g. hacking out over hilly terrain helps to develop and strengthen the muscles and teach balance; negotiating natural obstacles – branches, boggy ground, ditches etc. encourages co-ordination and an ability to place feet (hooves) carefully.

Avoid over facing keen horses and continue to promote confidence by always competing at a level below the standard being achieved in training at home.

The Rider:

Just as the show jumping horse will improve through working on flatwork skills, the show jumping rider will also benefit from the type of exercises prescribed for the dressage rider. A secure, balanced and effective position must first be established on the flat before progressing to riding over fences. By referring back to the individual components of fitness detailed in Chapter One, we can determine which areas are of most significance to the show jumping rider.

Aerobic Endurance:
Although many courses will be ridden against the clock and some will take only a few minutes to complete, the rider still needs a good level of

cardiovascular fitness to cope with the constant changing of position in the saddle as well as controlling the pace of the horse.

Anaerobic / Muscular Endurance:
No real need for anaerobic or muscular endurance in the show jumping rider.

Strength:
As with other disciplines, pure strength is unnecessary but a degree of strength is required to maintain a jumping position in the saddle and to control balance when changing from an upright seat to a forward seat. This will involve stability in the abdominal and back muscles, therefore core strength is essential.

Speed:
The rider has no need to train his muscles for pure speed, although he will need to be able to move quickly from one position to another.

Power:
Not an essential component of fitness for riding.

Body Composition:
Excessive body fat will potentially encroach on the rider's ability to move freely in the saddle. Due to the possibility of missing a take-off stride and consequently being 'left behind' or landing heavily on the saddle after a fence, a fatter rider must accept that this will undoubtedly create extra strain on the horse's muscles.

Flexibility:
A vital component of fitness for riding in all disciplines. The show jumping rider must develop the ability to sit into the saddle to control the speed between fences and also the ability to 'feel' a stride and go with the horse on take-off. Developing flexibility will enhance these skills and also allow the rider greater freedom to change position frequently from an upright position to a jumping position. The rider must be flexible enough to maintain his own balance through such movements without interfering with the balance and movement of his horse.

Show Jumping Rider Exercises:
The following exercises are designed to promote overall aerobic fitness and the strength and flexibility skills required to ride well over fences. Begin by practising the exercises to get a feel for the movement and then try to perform ten repetitions of each one. Focus on feeling the targeted muscle

group working in each case and then gradually increase the number of repetitions (up to twenty) to progress at your own pace. Always warm up gently before asking your muscles to work to avoid injury. *See* Chapter Ten – *Warm Up Routines* – for more information.

> **Tips:** building a course or moving jumps around before riding will provide an ideal warm-up session for your own body before exercising.

> **Note:** a guide to the location and function of the muscles can be found at the end of Chapter One.

Front Lunges: to stretch the hip flexors and strengthen the quadricep muscles - (*see* pictures 16a and 16b)
- Stand facing the bale with your feet hip-width apart
- Lunge forwards to step onto the bale with your right foot – use a yard broom for balance
- Bend your left knee and aim it towards the ground as you allow your left heel to lift from the ground
- Continue to gently lower your left knee until you feel a stretch down the front of your left thigh – hold for a few seconds
- Push back with your right foot to return to the start position

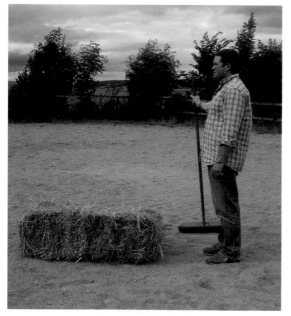

16a Front lunges

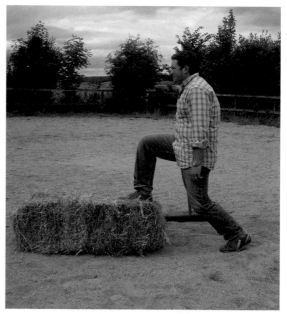

16b Front lunge with right leg

• Repeat the exercise using your left foot on the bale – then continue to alternate legs until you have completed ten lunges with each one
• Standing further back from the bale at the start will intensify the exercise
• Keep good posture, breathe out as you stretch each time and in as you push back

Forward Seat Squats: to stretch the adductor muscles and to strengthen the leg muscles – quadriceps, hamstrings, gluteals, calves. The back and shoulder muscles will also work when lifting the weight (*see* pictures 17a and 17b)

Tips: begin with a pair of jump cups (or similar weight) and then add more to increase the intensity when ready.

• Stand over the bale with your toes pointing slightly outwards
• Keep your knees relaxed and hold the jump cups in both hands in front of you
• Squat down as if aiming to sit on a chair behind you – stick your bottom out but keep your knees in line with your toes
• Keep good posture by keeping your head and neck in line with your spine

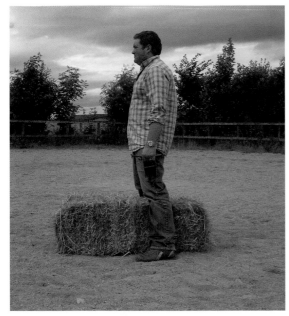

17a Forward seat squats

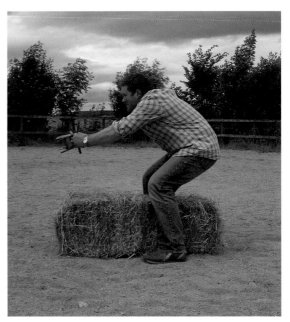

17b Squat down and raise your arms

- Raise your arms – keep a slight bend in your elbows – out in front of you and up to shoulder height as you squat down
- Breathe out through your mouth as you squat and hold the lowest position for a few seconds
- Breathe in through your nose as you stand up to relax your arms back to the start position
- Continue to repeat the whole exercise until you have completed ten squats

Side Shuttles: to work the heart and lungs (*see* pictures 18a and 18b)

> **Tips:** shorten the distance of the shuttles and work at speed to increase the intensity.

- Skip sideways, up on your toes, for five steps to the right
- Bend your knees and reach down to touch your right toes with your right hand

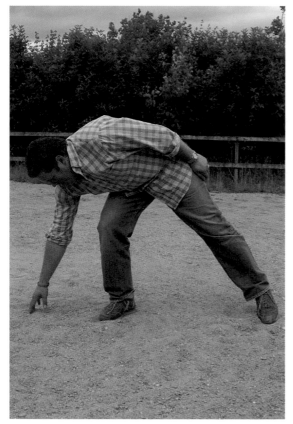 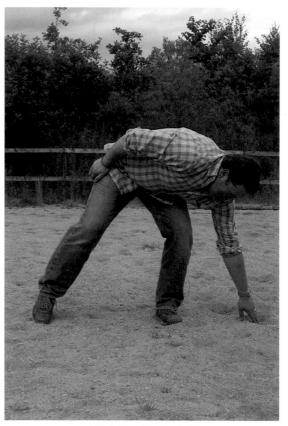

18a Side shuttle right   *18b Side shuttle left*

- Skip sideways, up on your toes, for five steps to the left
- Bend your knees and reach down to touch your left toes with your left hand
- Repeat until you have touched your toes ten times in total
- Stay relaxed, keep good posture as you skip and breathe normally – expect your breathing rate and heart rate to go up quite rapidly!

Tummy Tucks: to strengthen the abdominal muscles and work the hip flexors (*see* pictures 19a and 19b)

> **Tips:** to intensify this exercise, try straightening your leg out each time instead of lowering it and then try moving both legs together instead of individually – the muddier your boots are, the harder this will feel!

- Lie back on the bale with your head and neck supported as in the picture
- Lift both feet up from the ground to form a 90 degree angle with knees bent – place your hands on the edge of the bale for support

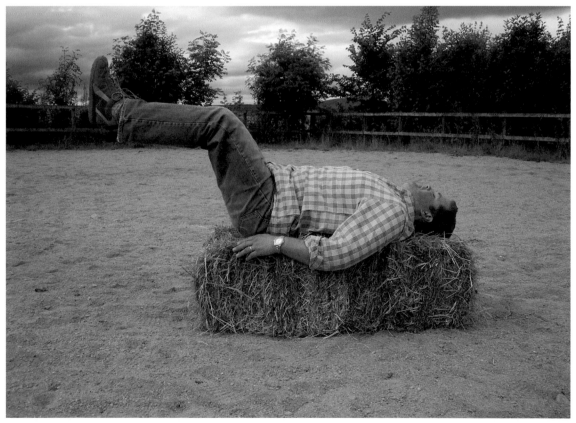

19a Tummy tucks

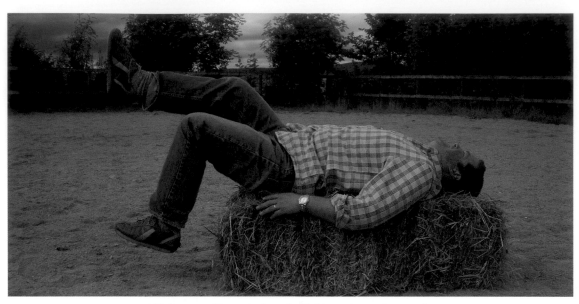

19b Lower alternate legs to tighten stomach muscles

- Lower your right leg slowly towards the ground until you feel your stomach muscles tighten – breathe out through your mouth and hold for a few seconds
- Breathe in through your nose as you return your right leg to the start position and then repeat the exercise using your left leg
- Continue to use alternate legs until you have lowered each leg ten times
- Keep a neutral (relaxed) spine position on the bale

To add some fun to your exercise sessions, try creating your own *'Jumping Circuit'* in the arena. Utilise the time spent building a course or moving the jumps around to warm up your muscles and then jog or power walk your way around the course completing a combination of the above exercises and those learned in Chapter Two along the way. Begin by performing the exercises at each fence for thirty seconds and then, as you get fitter, try to keep going for a whole minute each time.

Jumping Circuit

Fence One:
Alternate arm circles – see Chapter Two.

Fence Two:
Side stretches – see Chapter Two.

Fence Three:
> Front lunges – without the bale (or use a jump filler if stable enough to support your weight).

Fence Four:
> Side shuttles – skip for five steps each way, or less if you'd like to make it harder!

Fence Five:
> Trunk rotation – see Chapter Two – instead of using a lunge whip just hold your arms out to each side at shoulder height.

Fence Six:
> Heel kicks – jog on the spot and kick your heels up towards your bottom.

Fence Seven:
> Forward seat squats – without the bale.

Fence Eight:
> Toe touch jumps – keep your feet together and bend your knees to reach down and touch your toes. Jump up in the air as you straighten up and reach for the sky – then continue to repeat.

Fence Nine:
> Hip swings – see Chapter Two – remember to swap legs at the half-way point!

Fence Ten:
> Walk around the fence to lower your heart and breathing rate if they feel high. Whole body stretch – bend your knees to touch your toes and then breathe in deeply as you stand up and reach for the sky with both arms. Breathe out as you relax and repeat twice more.

Aim to exercise at least two or three times each week. The above exercises can be used in conjunction with those learned in Chapters Two and Three to create your own training programme. Make use of a variety of exercises to suit your own circumstances and focus on those which are of most benefit to you at your current level of fitness – suggestions are provided in Chapter Twelve. If you expect your horse to give you a clear round each time you compete, then it seems only fair that you should put the same degree of effort into improving your own fitness in order to help rather than hinder.

Case Study:

Rider – Alex Clements
Age – 47

Riding Experience:

Alex runs his own livery yard and has ridden since childhood. He trains his clients' horses and competes regularly in affiliated show jumping events on his own two youngsters so he rides an average of four hours each day with one day off each week after a competition.

Alex admits to feeling less supple than he once did and finds that a day in the saddle leaves him feeling tired. As he rides a variety of horses, he is aware that his own lack of flexibility may limit his ability to relax into the saddle and gel with the natural movement of each horse. The following programme was designed to increase Alex's general aerobic fitness in order to boost his energy levels and also to restore his flexibility through regular stretching.

Saturday:

Competition day – an average of two classes on each of his own horses.

Sunday:

1. No riding but all normal yard duties.
2. Long soak in the bath followed by the advanced stretches detailed in Chapter Ten – lying hamstring, adductor, lower back and gluteal, and hip flexor stretches.

Monday:

1. Mucking out etc. to warm up, followed by a ten minute (gradually building up to twenty minutes) power walk / jog.
2. Training / exercising of horses – average of four hours:
Before the first ride – all joint mobility exercises detailed in Chapter Four – neck, elbows, wrists, trunk / spine, hips / pelvis, knees and ankles plus all the flexibility exercises detailed in Chapter Two – shoulder shrugs, arm circles, side stretches, trunk rotation and hip swings.
After each ride – all daily stretches for upper and lower body (Chapter Ten).

Tuesday:
1. Mucking out / grooming etc. to warm up.
2. The Jumping Circuit – one minute on each exercise.
3. Schooling of horses:
After each schooling session – daily stretches for upper and lower body (Chapter Ten).

Wednesday:
As Monday.

Thursday:
1. All normal yard duties plus riding.
2. After a long soak in the bath, all advanced stretches – as Sunday.

Friday:
1. Mucking out / grooming etc. to warm up muscles.
2. All flexibilty exercises as Monday.
3. Power walk / jog of at least ten minutes.
After jog – all daily stretches for upper and lower body (Chapter Ten).
4. Ride as normal.

Summary of Rider Fitness Training for Show Jumping:
- Train for aerobic endurance to prevent fatigue
- Train for flexibility to be able to move easily in the saddle
- Train for core strength to be able to maintain balance through changes of position and pace
- A supple rider will be a better balanced, lighter and more effective rider

EVENTING

This is an extremely demanding sport for both horse and rider so both parties must be physically and mentally fit for the challenge. It takes many years of preparation to ensure that a horse has developed sufficient strength and fitness to deal with the physical challenges involved and also the maturity to cope with the very individual stresses created by each

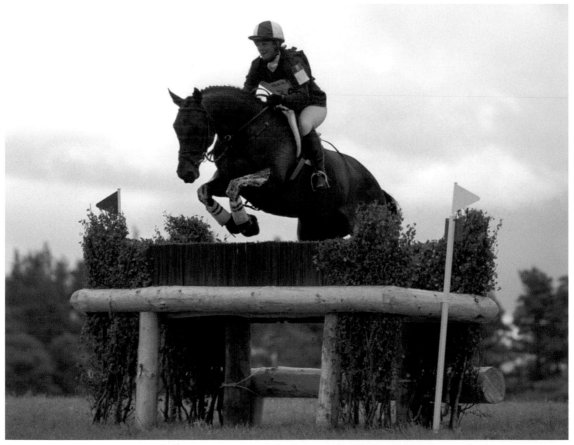

Both parties must have faith in each other's abilities

element of an event. The rider must devote just as much time to preparing themselves if a successful partnership is to be formed and both parties must have faith in each other's abilities to be able to compete safely and with confidence. The rider must be every bit as fit as the horse, because an unfit rider will not be able to help their horse when the going gets tough.

The Horse:

Whether aiming to compete in a one-, two-, or three-day-event it is clear that the eventing horse must be physically fit to cope with the demands of three very different disciplines. He must possess all the skills already outlined in the chapters on the dressage horse and the show jumping horse plus he must be able to complete all of the tasks presented to him in the cross-country phase. Similar to British Dressage and BSJA, graded levels of competition exist within British Eventing to provide a means of progression for both horse and rider. Newcomers to the sport begin with the Introductory classes and then progress through Pre-Novice to Novice and on to Intermediate, then Advanced. To be able to upgrade, both horse and rider must have a proven track record in competition at the existing level before being permitted to enter at the next level. This is an extremely effective way of limiting the dangers of the sport and ensures that both parties are better prepared for the physical and mental demands of each event.

In a one-day-event, the horse performs in all three disciplines – dressage, cross-country and show jumping – in the same day. In a two-day-event, the dressage and show jumping phases are held on the first day, with an extended cross-country phase on the second day. In a three-day-event, the dressage is held on the first day, then cross-country on the second day and show jumping on the third day. This level of eventing is considered to be the ultimate test of fitness and stamina in the horse as suppleness, energy and obedience are all necessary to compete.

A horse must be a minimum of five years old to compete and, once at Novice level, must be a minimum height of 148 centimetres (14.2 hands). The degree of difficulty in the dressage phase increases at each level. There is also an increase in the height and width of fences in the show jumping phase and the time limit in which to complete the course decreases. The same applies to the cross-country obstacles where technical difficulty increases along with height and width. The courses become longer and more jumping efforts are required but the time limit in which to complete the phase again decreases. At Advanced level, the cross-country course may be as long as four kilometres (two and a half miles) and as many as forty jumping efforts could be included. Bear in mind that a horse at this level will still need to be obedient enough to perform in the dressage arena before being able to 'let off steam' in the cross-country phase, yet remain energetic and supple enough to complete a course of show jumps afterwards.

The event horse is undoubtedly an all-round athlete and could be likened to a human triathlete. In a one-day competition, the horse will be afforded a minimum of thirty minutes rest between each of the three phases but the triathlete must actually continue straight from the swim phase to the cycle and on to the run without a break. In both cases, equine and human, success will come to the athlete who performs well in all three disciplines so the training programme must address areas of weakness, as well as natural strengths, in order to produce a balanced performance.

Top Training Tips from Event Riders:
Focus on achieving a good level of base fitness before introducing specific training for individual elements.

Aim for uniformity of performance in all three elements at your level of competition before progressing in any individual one i.e. train weak areas to match strengths.

Take time to build fitness gradually and progressively.

The Rider:

At all levels of competition, the event rider must be every bit as fit as the event horse if they are to become a successful partnership. However, I have often witnessed riders collapse into flushed and breathless heaps as they return from the cross-country phase. How can an unfit rider possibly help their horse to tackle the enormously demanding task of competing in such an arduous sport? The answer is simple: they can't! In my opinion it is the responsibility of every rider who wishes to take part in eventing to ensure that they, not just their horse, are physically fit for the sport. By looking at the components of fitness introduced in Chapter One, we can see which areas are most relevant to the event rider.

Aerobic Endurance:
An essential component of fitness for the event rider due to the duration of most competitions. Energy levels must be maintained from start to finish as it's towards the end of an event that the horse will require the most help

from the rider. Imagine yourself taking part in an all-day, or even multi-day, hill walk with a backpack that constantly becomes heavier and more awkward to carry with each step.

Anaerobic / Muscular Endurance:
Not essential to the event rider.

Strength:
As with the other disciplines, core strength is essential to be able to maintain a correct riding position. The cross-country phase of an event will be ridden in jumping or galloping position so a greater degree of leg strength must be developed to promote a secure, balanced and effective 'seat'.

Speed:
The rider has no need to develop speed in their own training.

Power:
Not an essential component of fitness for the rider.

Body Composition:
Excessive body fat brings with it many health concerns that may restrict the rider's ability to train effectively for event riding. Extra body weight gained through stored fat, as opposed to lean tissue, will place further strain on the heart and lungs when training the cardiovascular system to improve aerobic endurance. Restricted movement around the joints could also impede the rider's ability to move freely in the saddle. This creates problems when negotiating cross-country terrain as the rider must be supple and mobile enough to manoeuvre quickly into the best position to balance themselves and their horse.

Flexibility:
An essential component of fitness for the rider. Flexibility is needed in all areas of event riding if the rider is to remain secure in the saddle and in a position to help themselves and their horse to avoid fatigue.

Event Rider Exercises:
The power walking / jogging programme contained in Chapter Three – *The Next Step* – should be followed in order to develop improved aerobic endurance. Once able to jog for ten minutes, the target should then become a jog of four kilometres (two and a half miles) over undulating terrain. If the thought of such a distance horrifies you, bear in mind that this is potentially the distance you will expect your horse to carry you and

he will have up to forty jumping efforts to contend with too. I'd say you've still got the better deal!

Aerobic Endurance Training:

A jog of four kilometres (two and a half miles) over undulating and perhaps muddy terrain will take around thirty minutes to complete. Develop the ability to jog for ten minutes, as explained in Chapter Three, and then continue to add an extra two minutes of jogging (or power walking) to each session. Don't be tempted to add too much too soon, remember that your body needs time to adapt, and progressive training is needed in order to achieve long-term improvement safely.

> **Tips:** stretch the leg muscles at the end of each jogging session (*see* Chapter Ten - daily stretches / lower body).

Strength Training Exercises:

The following exercises are designed to work specifically on the areas of most importance to the event rider. Aim to do the exercises three times a week but remember the importance of warming up the muscles thoroughly before asking them to work.

> **Note:** a guide to the location and function of the muscles can be found at the end of Chapter One.

Step-Ups: to work the heart, lungs and leg muscles – quadriceps, gluteals and calves (*see* pictures 20a, 20b and 20c)

> **Tips:** increase the speed of the movements to intensify the exercise.

• Stand facing the bale and then step up using your right leg to lead the way
• Step up with your left foot so that both feet are on the bale
• Step back to the ground with your right foot first, followed by your left foot
• Repeat the exercise to complete twenty step-ups – right leg leading for ten then left leg leading for ten
• Keep good posture, use your arms to assist the stepping action, breathe normally but work at a speed that raises your heart rate

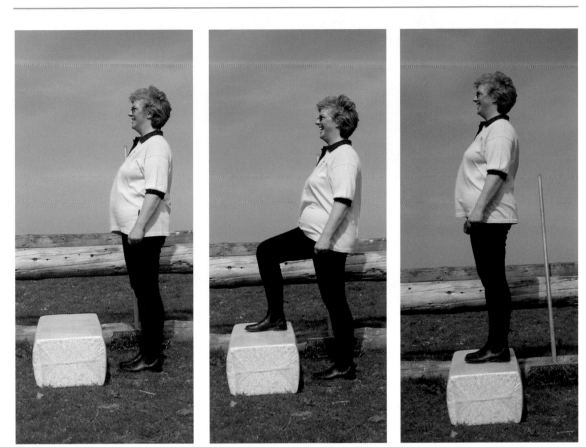

20a Step-ups

20b Step up using right leg

20c Step up with left leg to complete the move

Jack Knives: to work the abdominal muscles including obliques (*see* pictures 21a and 21b overleaf)

Tips: use your available hand to support the weight of your head to avoid neck strain developing.

• Lie back with your head and neck supported by the bale and keep both feet on the ground
• Allow your arms to swing backwards behind you to feel a stretch in your stomach muscles
• Swing your right arm and raise your left leg simultaneously to meet in the air directly over your body – aim to touch your left toes with your right fingers – breathe out through your mouth

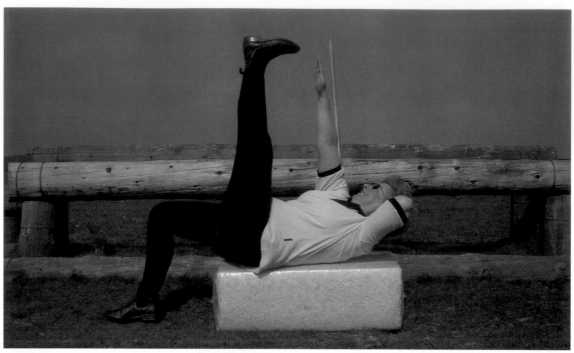

21a Swing right arm to meet left leg

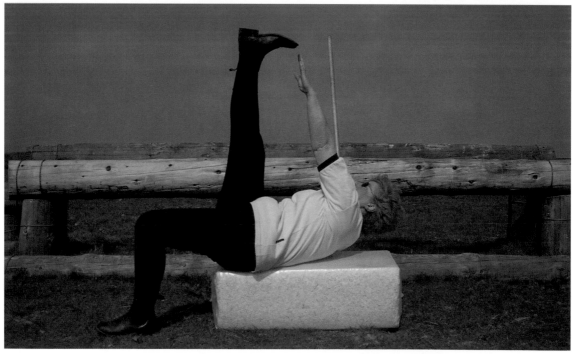

21b Swing left arm to meet right leg

• Breathe in through your nose as you relax back to the start position and then repeat the exercise using your left arm and right leg
• Continue to alternate arms and legs until you have completed twenty movements – don't worry if you can't reach your toes every time!
• Keep your spine relaxed on the bale (avoid arching), take your time and feel a stretch in the stomach muscles as you breathe in each time

Standing Push-Ups: to work the pectoral muscles and triceps (*see* pictures 22a and 22b)

> **Tips:** you can advance this exercise by using something lower than the wall e.g. a bale, jump filler or mounting block.

• Stand facing a wall (or something solid) and place your hands against it at shoulder height and width apart
• Lean in towards the wall by bending your elbows – imagine you are aiming to touch the wall with your nose – breathe in through your nose

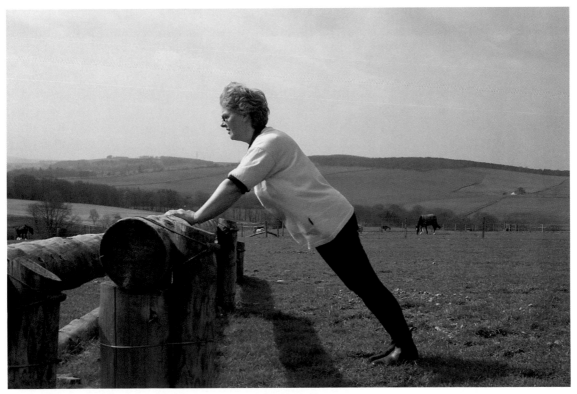

22a Standing push-ups

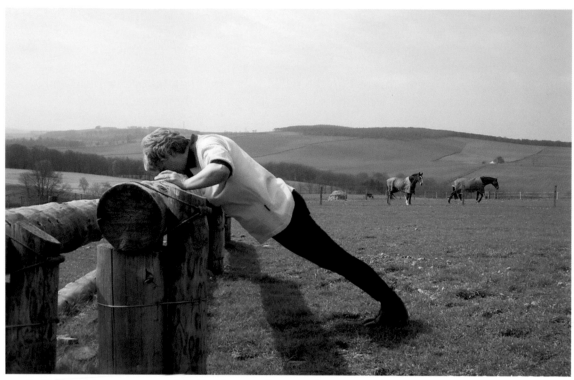

22b Bend your elbows to lower your body

• Push back with your arms to return to the start position – breathe out through your mouth
• Continue to repeat the whole exercise until you have completed ten push ups
• Keep good posture in your back – the further away from the wall you stand at the start, the more intense the exercise becomes

Jockey Squats: to strengthen the legs – quadriceps, knee joint and ankle joint – and improve the ability to 'hold' a jumping position – (*see* picture 23)

Tips: the 90 degree angle in your knees is very important – if you don't squat low enough or you actually squat too low, you are effectively cheating!

• Lean back against any object solid enough to support your weight comfortably
• Position yourself as if sitting on an imaginary chair and form a 90 degree angle in your knee joints

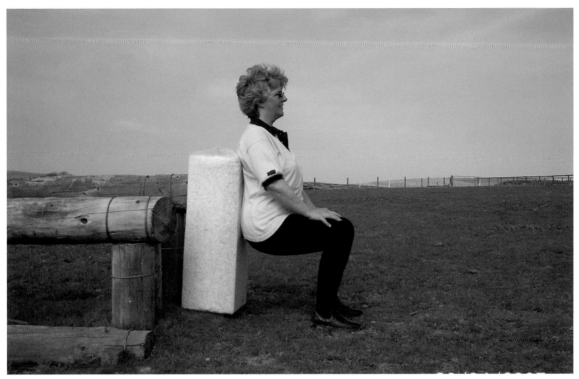

23 Jockey squats

• Hold this position for one minute – you may need to stand up from time to time to rest
• Do not put pressure with your hands on your legs (leaning on your thighs puts pressure on the working muscles) and breathe normally.

Grooming Kit Lifts: to strengthen the back and arm muscles – lats, rhomboids and biceps (*see* pictures 24a and 24b overleaf)

> **Tips:** start with a light grooming kit to get the feel of the exercise and then add more items to increase the weight when you feel ready.

• Position yourself on the bale with left knee and hand in line under left hip and shoulder
• Keep your right foot on the ground for balance
• Pick up the grooming kit with your right hand and lift it towards your shoulder – breathe out through your mouth as you lift
• Lower it slowly towards the ground again but repeat the lift without allowing it to rest on the ground – breathe in through your nose as you lower

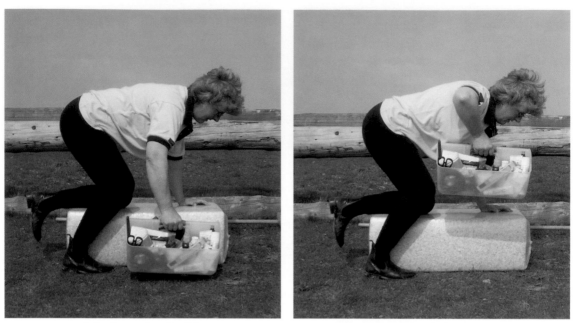

24a Grooming kit lifts   *24b Begin with a light grooming kit*

• Keep your back flat with head, neck and spine in line
• Repeat to complete ten lifts with your right arm before changing positions to complete ten lifts using your left arm

Back Extensions: to work the lower back muscles (*see* pictures 25a and 25b)

Tips: this exercise could be replaced by the 'plank' exercise (Chapter Two) if preferred.

• Lie face down on the bale as far forwards as possible but keep both feet (toes) on the ground for balance
• Place your fingers on your temples and begin to raise your head and shoulders gently by recruiting your back muscles – this is only a small move
• Keep your head and neck in line with your spine (continue to look down at the ground) to avoid straining your neck – hold the raised position for ten seconds
• Return to the start position and allow your back muscles to relax before repeating
• Breathe normally throughout and keep your feet on the ground

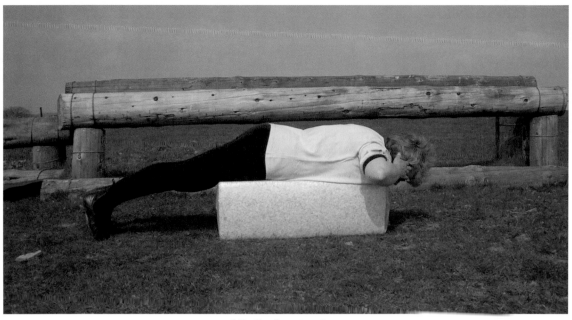

25a Back extensions

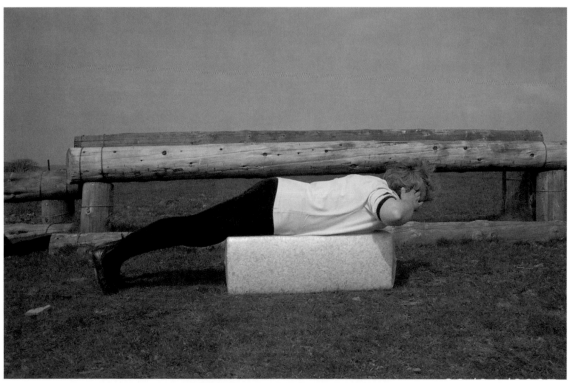

25b Raise your head and shoulders

Flexibility Exercises:

The flexibility exercises learned in Chapter Two – *Base Fitness Training* – should still be used regularly to help maintain joint mobility. The following exercises are designed to provide alternatives and to encourage an increase in the range of movement where appropriate.

Posture Stretch: to stretch the adductor muscles and the upper body – abdominals, obliques, lower back, lats, biceps and triceps (*see* pictures 26a and 26b)

> **Tips:** the further apart you place your feet, the more intense the stretch becomes.

- Stand astride the bale with your toes turned out slightly and keep your knees relaxed
- Start with your arms hanging by your sides and then raise them out to the side and up overhead as you lower your bottom towards the bale
- Keep an upright posture by remaining tall in your upper body and squatting straight down (avoid sticking your bottom out!)
- Breathe out through your mouth as you squat down and stretch – feel the stretch on the inside of your thighs, the sides of your body, stomach, back, and arms as you reach up – hold for a few seconds
- Breathe in through your nose as you relax back to the start position
- Repeat twice more – move slowly and focus on correct posture

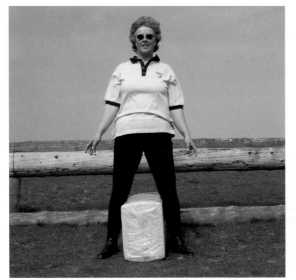
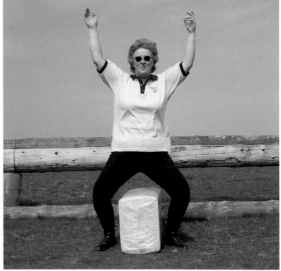

26a Posture stretch   *26b Squat down and stretch*

Advanced Hip Swings: to loosen the hip joints and surrounding muscles – gluteals and hip flexors (*see* pictures 27a, 27b, 27c and 27d)

Tips: your range of movement will increase as you practise so start sensibly and avoid forcing any movement.

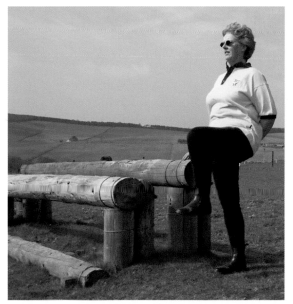

27a Advanced hip swings

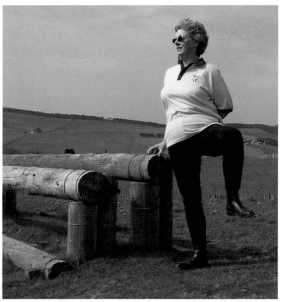

27b Rotate leg outwards

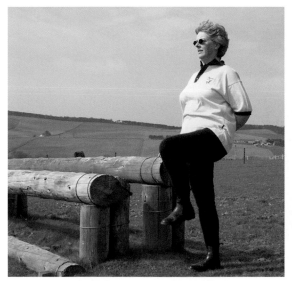

27c Return to start position

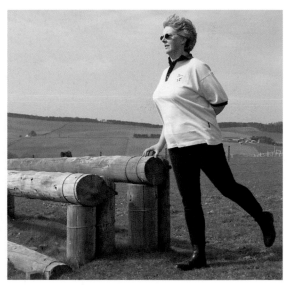

27d Swing leg backwards

• Lean against something secure for balance and stand on one leg (relaxed knee)
• Raise your other leg in front of you by bending your knee – exactly as in the 'hip swings' exercise learned in Chapter Two
• From the raised position, swing your leg outwards away from your body as wide as possible – remain facing forwards and aim to keep your knee up at hip height
• Return your leg towards your body and then allow it to swing gently behind you (as in the hip swing exercise)
• Complete ten movements with each leg individually
• Keep good posture, move slowly and breathe normally

Torso Twist: to stretch the trunk muscles – abdominals, obliques and lower back (*see* pictures 28a, 28b and 28c)

> **Tips:** this exercise could also be done without the bale.

• Stand astride the bale with toes turned out slightly and knees relaxed (slightly bent)
• Hold your arms out at shoulder height on each side of your body

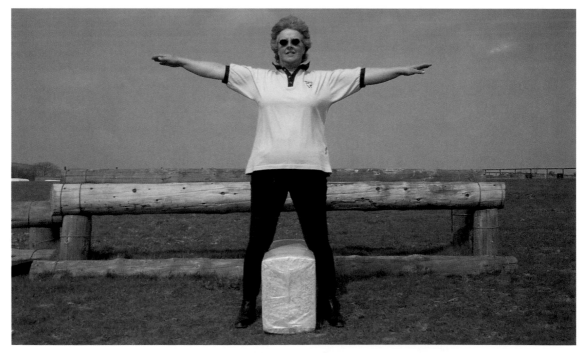

28a Torso twist

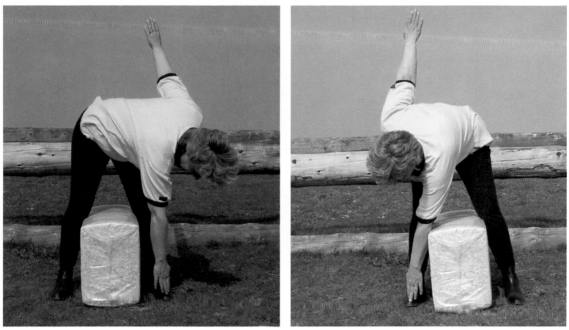

28b Twist right arm to left toe   *28c Twist left arm to right toe*

• Twist through your waist to the right, as far as possible – maintain shoulder height with your arm position
• Return to the start position and then stretch down to touch your left toes with your right fingers
• Return to the start position – arms still shoulder height – and then repeat the whole exercise twisting to the left this time
• Continue to alternate sides until you have twisted and stretched each way ten times
• Breathe in through your nose as you twist to the side and out through your mouth as you reach for your toes each time
• Keep your knees relaxed to avoid stress on the joints – don't worry if you can't reach your toes every time!

The above exercises can be used in conjunction with those used to improve fitness for dressage and show jumping in Chapters Five and Six. It is important to create a fitness training programme that fits in with other elements of your daily routine and also a programme of exercises that is suitable for your current level of fitness as this will make the best use of valuable time – *see* Chapter Twelve for suggestions. Training a horse for eventing takes considerable time but remember that as little as ten minutes of effort from you each day can go a long way towards improving your own fitness for eventing.

Case Study:

Rider – Sally Brodie
Age – 28

Riding Experience:

Sally rode as a child and then competed regularly in eventing until the age of twenty-three when she gave up riding to start a family. After a four-year break and two children later, she returned to riding with a view to competing her homebred young horse in Introductory and then Novice events. The following programme was designed to improve Sally's general aerobic fitness and to increase her core strength and flexibility in preparation for riding competitively. Sally works on a part-time, freelance basis so on days when she had other commitments, she exercised / stretched early in the morning and rode in the evening.

Saturday:
1.   Long hack incorporating twenty minutes of leading in hand – split into two ten-minute sessions – on route.
2.   All daily stretches detailed in Chapter Ten – upper body and lower body.

Sunday:
1.   No riding as this will become a rest day when the competition season starts.
2.   After a soak in the bath, all advanced stretches detailed in Chapter Ten – lying hamstring, adductor, lower back and gluteal, and hip flexor.

Monday:
1.   Morning:
Normal riding routine of at least one hour.
2.   Afternoon:
Warm up with ten minutes of power walking or jogging around the field to check on the horses, followed by all event rider exercises.
All daily stretches (Chapter Ten).

Tuesday:
1. Morning:
Warm up by grooming etc. for at least ten minutes.
All flexibility exercises detailed in Chapter Two – shoulder shrugs, arm circles, side stretches and hip swings.
2. Afternoon:
Twenty minute brisk walk / jog with children in buggy.
All daily stretches (Chapter Ten).

Wednesday:
1. Morning:
Hack out incorporating at least ten minutes of leading in hand on route.
All daily stretches (Chapter Ten).
2. Evening:
Long soak in the bath followed by all advanced stretches (Chapter Ten).

Thursday.
As Monday.

Friday:
As Tuesday.

Summary of Rider Fitness Training for Eventing:
• Train for aerobic endurance to prevent fatigue
• Train for core stability and flexibility to create a secure, mobile and effective position in the saddle
• Stretch regularly to maintain flexibility and to reduce the risk of injury
• Advance your own fitness level as your horse progresses in training and in competition

CHAPTER EIGHT
ENDURANCE

Top level endurance riding is a tough, demanding sport but even at the very beginning of a competitive career both horse and rider must be fit for their chosen distance. The welfare of the horse is of paramount importance at all levels and the sport promotes this by including vet checks at various stages to monitor the horse's condition. Unfortunately, such checks are not mandatory for the riders! Endurance riding requires skill and good horsemanship just like any other equestrian sport but, unlike most other

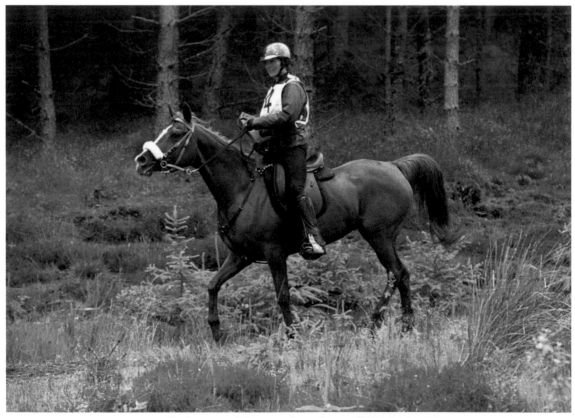

Endurance riding can be a demanding sport

disciplines, the continuous time spent in the saddle will amount to hours rather than minutes. One single ride will generally involve several different types of terrain and often several changes of weather, so no amount of expensive equipment will protect the horse from an unfit, unbalanced rider who places unacceptable stress and strain on the horse's body by sitting badly in the saddle – hour after hour! Riders must have a thorough understanding of the importance of changing trot diagonals frequently to help distribute their weight evenly across the horse's body and the need to ensure that the horse is able to use both leading legs in canter equally to maintain symmetry and balance.

The Horse:

When planning to compete in endurance riding events under Endurance GB rules, (Scottish Endurance Riding Club rules vary slightly), the starting point for most is to take part in a Pleasure Ride. These are sometimes called training or social rides and are open to horses from four years old and can be of any distance up to 32 kilometres (20 miles). Speed parameters are in place to ensure a sensible minimum and maximum time limit for the route so the optimum pace will be economical. The next level of competition includes Set Speed Rides and Graded Rides which are usually between 30 and 80 kilometres (18 and 50 miles) in length but the horse must be a minimum of five years of age to take part in this category of events. A novice horse is not permitted to take part in any more than ten rides in its first season and cannot compete at advanced level until at least its second season. Advanced horse and rider combinations can take part in Endurance Rides that generally range from 65 to 160 kilometres (40 to 100 miles) in a day or even further over several days but the horse must be a minimum of seven years old to compete at this level. So, progressing from novice to advanced level may require at least four years of specific training and for many competing at top level this process will have taken considerably longer.

Horses and ponies of any breed and of all shapes and sizes can take part in long-distance riding events as there are generally no restrictions in terms of height. As with other disciplines, certain types feature regularly at top level and in this case the predominant breed is the pure-bred, or part-bred, Arabian. At all levels, good conformation and smooth paces are important to help limit fatigue in both parties and compact, lighter framed horses are favoured over heavier breeds for the faster events. A level-headed temperament will also help the horse to cope with the mental stresses of competition and will make the whole journey, whether training or competing, much more enjoyable for both horse and rider. However, the only

Body Composition:
The ability to ride 'light' will undoubtedly help the horse in his task. Excess body fat serves no useful purpose so it only adds to the horse's burden by placing extra stress on the heart, lungs and limbs.

Flexibility:
This is the most important component of fitness for all riders. Being able to move freely with the horse helps to prevent fatigue in long-distance events and developing a better 'feel' in the saddle will allow for better pace judgement in timed rides where it is important to be able to maintain an economical, rhythmical pace to save energy.

Endurance Rider Exercises:
The training programme detailed in Chapter Three – *The Next Step* – provides a means of improving cardiovascular fitness by jogging or power walking. The most effective way to continue developing further without encroaching on valuable fitness training time needed for your horse is to incorporate your own training into your allocated riding time.

Aerobic Endurance Training:
Every hour of riding time given to you by your horse should be matched by ten minutes of jogging or power walking effort – on your own two feet! So, if you are going to ride your horse for a total of four hours over the course of a week, you should be prepared to jog or power walk for a total of forty minutes in that same week. To prevent this from becoming prohibitively time consuming it makes sense to combine the fitness training for both rider and horse into the same session. During a one hour ride, dismount and walk or jog with your horse for ten minutes – this could be broken down into several shorter jogs spread out over the duration of the ride e.g. five separate jogs of two minutes each time or two jogs of five minutes. The amount of time you spend on the ground at any one time will be governed by the type of terrain you are riding over but the most practical approach is to dismount and jog or walk over areas of rough ground and on downhill sections. The main advantage of removing your weight from the saddle over this type of terrain is that the horse then only has to cope with maintaining his own balance without any interference from the rider thus ensuring that valuable energy is saved and the risk of injury is greatly reduced. Care must be taken to avoid injuring your own ankles over rough terrain but greater strength and flexibility will be achieved through practice. The additional effort of mounting and dismounting frequently throughout a ride will also help to prepare your muscles for the rigours of negotiating a common hazard on long rides – gates! – and your horse also gains a valuable lesson in manners by learning to stand still as you mount.

The following exercises are designed to help stretch and develop the muscles needed most by the endurance rider. They should be used in conjunction with the exercises already learned in Chapter Two to create a twenty-minute stable yard workout and practised at least three times a week.

> **Tips:** always warm up your muscles before asking them to work, *see* Chapter Ten – *Warm Up Routines for Riders*.

Stretching and Strengthening Exercises:

The muscles of the legs – calves, hamstrings, quadriceps, adductors, hip flexors and gluteals – must be both strong and supple to cope with long periods of sustained effort, particularly in rising trot, without becoming fatigued as a tired rider will become a much heavier rider. This also applies to the core stability muscles – abdominals, obliques and back – as without strength and flexibility in the trunk, the rider will lack postural control and will be unable to sit lightly in the saddle or move easily with the movement of the horse. An uncomfortable rider will very quickly create an uncomfortable horse!

> **Note:** a guide to the location and function of the muscles can be found at the end of Chapter One.

Leg Ups: to condition the leg muscles – hip flexors, glutes, quadriceps and calves – and to work the heart and lungs (*see* pictures 29a, 29b and 29c)

> **Tips:** any solid item can be used in place of the bale – use a low 'step' to begin with and then go higher to increase the intensity when ready.

- Place your right foot on the bale leaving your left foot on the ground
- Bend both knees to crouch slightly – allow your left heel to lift from the ground
- Spring up on to the bale by pushing off the ground with your left toes then immediately return your left foot to the ground
- Continue repeating the exercise to complete ten quick movements using the same leg and then swap positions to perform ten more using the other leg
- Keep good posture (avoid swinging your upper body) and breathe normally – expect your heart rate and breathing rate to go up!

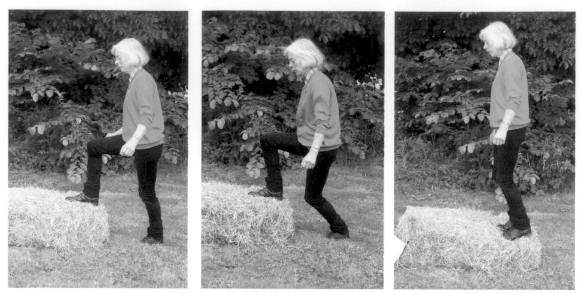

29a Leg ups   *29b Crouch down*   *29c Spring up*

Hop Overs: to condition the muscles used when mounting and dismounting – lower back, glutes, adductors, quadriceps and calves – and to work the heart and lungs (*see* pictures 30a, 30b and 30c)

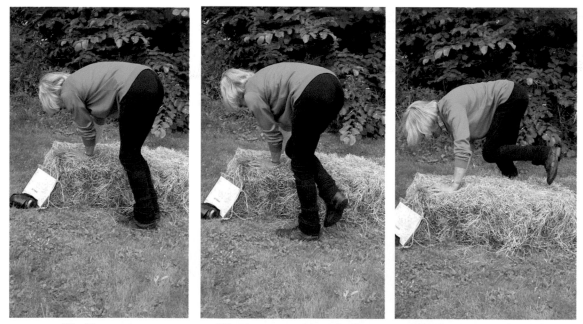

30a Hop overs   *30b Hop over with right foot*   *30c Hop over with left foot*

Tips: use a higher platform to increase the intensity or keep both feet together when 'hopping' over the bale.

- Stand to the side of the bale and bend down to place both hands on the top – keep a slight bend in your elbows
- Hop over the bale, one foot at a time, to arrive on the other side
- Repeat the movements to hop back over to the starting side then continue 'hopping' until both feet have crossed over the bale twenty times
- Keep joints – elbows, knees, ankles – relaxed to avoid jarring and breathe normally

Girth Tightener: to strengthen the abdominal muscles including obliques – (*see* pictures 31a and 31b)

Tips: support the weight of your head with your spare hand to avoid neck strain.

- Lie back on the bale with your head supported
- Raise both feet straight in the air and cross your ankles

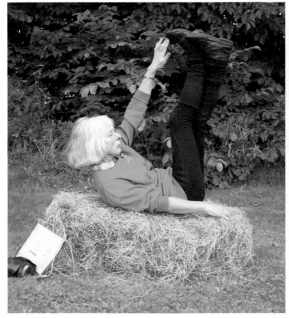
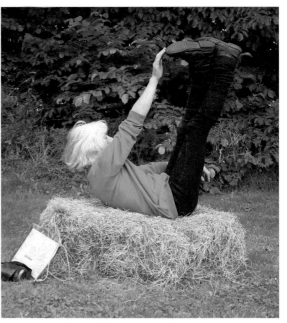

31a Girth tightener   *31b Reach up to touch your toes*

- Reach up with your right arm to touch your toes – keep your legs straight – breathe out through your mouth as you stretch
- Relax your shoulders back to the bale – breathe in through your nose – then immediately reach up with your left hand to touch your toes
- Continue to alternate hands until you have touched your toes twenty times
- Aim to move quickly but focus on using your stomach muscles as you reach up each time – keep your legs perpendicular to the ground

Superman Plank: to strengthen the core, postural – abdominal and back –muscles (*see* pictures 32a and 32b)

> **Tips:** practise 'the plank' exercise (Chapter Five) before progressing to this more advanced exercise.

- Position yourself on the bale with elbows under shoulders, and toes on the ground

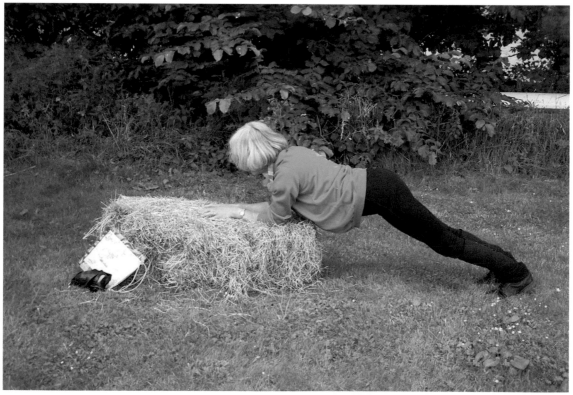

32a Form a plank with your body

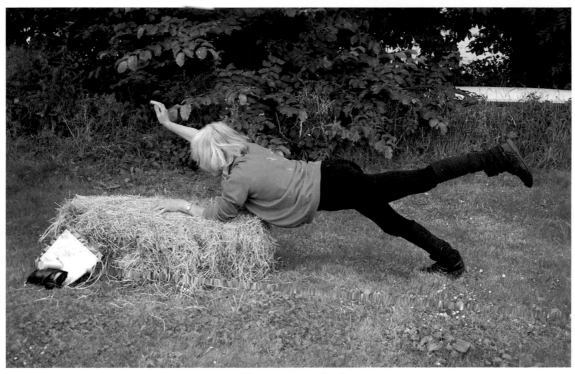

32b Superman plank

• Raise and straighten your right arm and left leg simultaneously – aim to hold for thirty seconds but don't worry if you wobble, it will take practise!
• Pull in your stomach muscles towards your spine but continue to breathe normally
• Relax back to the start position and repeat the exercise using your left arm and right leg for a further thirty seconds
• Keep your head and neck in line with your spine so that your body forms a 'plank'– sagging in the middle is cheating!
• Relax by placing your knees on the ground when necessary until you can complete an entire minute

Sumo Squats: to work the leg muscles – gluteals, hamstrings and quadriceps – and to increase flexibility around the hip joints and in the adductor muscles (*see* pictures 33a, 33b and 33c overleaf)

• Stand astride the bale with toes turned out slightly and knees relaxed
• Squat down as if about to sit on the bale - feel the stretch in the adductor muscles

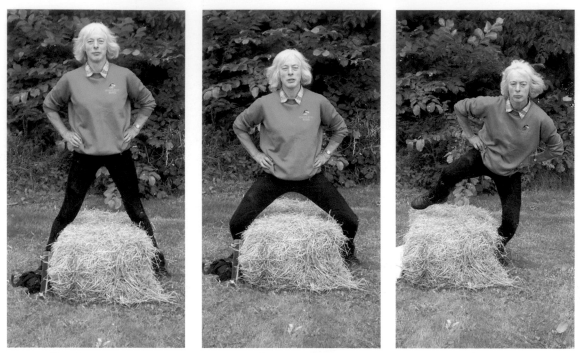

33a Sumo squats   33b Squat down   33c Transfer your weight

• Stand up and transfer your weight over on to your left leg while raising your right leg with hip and knee bent – like a sumo wrestler!
• Return to the squat position and then repeat the exercise using your other leg
• Continue to alternate legs until each leg has been raised ten times
• Take your time and breathe normally throughout

Twister: to work the heart and lungs and to improve flexibility and condition in the trunk muscles – abdominals, obliques, lats and lower back (*see* pictures 34a and 34b)

Tips: move quickly and jump higher to increase the intensity.

• Raise your hands to chest height and elbows to shoulder height
• Keep your feet together and a slight bend in your knees
• Make small jumps on the spot and twist from your waist by positioning your feet to the right then the left
• Continue to face forwards as you twist – allow your upper body to twist in the opposite direction to your feet

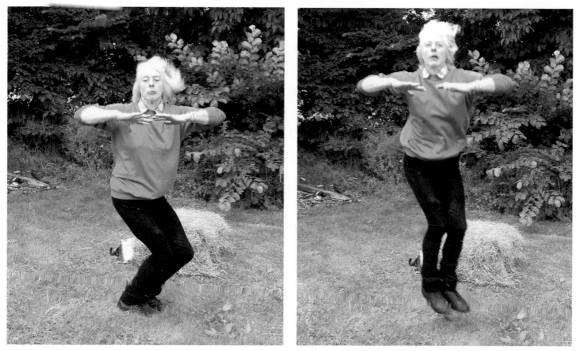

34a Twister   34b Make small jumps

- Keep your elbows up at shoulder height and keep knees and ankles relaxed to avoid jarring
- Aim to jump and twist for one minute – expect your heart rate and breathing rate to go up considerably!

The above exercises provide a means of improving fitness for endurance riding but they can only be of benefit if used to supplement a regular riding routine. Only by riding in long-distance events can the body truly become conditioned to cope with the demands of the sport. However, bad habits are easily formed in the saddle so the most effective way to prevent poor posture from limiting the rider's ability, and therefore making the horse's job harder, is to train the appropriate muscle groups when not actually in the saddle. It will also be of great benefit to both parties if the rider maintains at least a good base level of fitness during the off-season so as to lighten the load on the deconditioned horse's muscles when coming back into work. Fitness training for the rider can be continued throughout the year and will be particularly useful during the winter months when it's often too dark to fit in long rides. Further information is provided in Chapters Eleven and Twelve.

Case Study:

Rider - Kitty Sloan
Age - 60

Riding Experience:

Kitty has ridden since childhood and has always owned her own horse. She has never ridden competitively in any discipline and rides purely for pleasure. After joining in a Pleasure Ride organised by her local riding club, she decided to train seriously towards more competitive endurance events. The following programme was designed to improve Kitty's overall fitness in preparation for the many hours of riding and training needed to elevate her nine-year-old part-bred Arab from 'happy hacker' status up to the fitness required for a Graded Ride of up to 80 kms (50 miles). Kitty works as a school teacher so she used this programme during school holidays and then exercised early in the morning and rode in the evening after work during term time.

Saturday:
1. Long, steady hack to gradually increase mileage and/or time spent in the saddle.
2. Followed by all daily stretches detailed in Chapter Ten – pectorals, rhomboids, triceps, quadriceps, hamstrings and calves.

Sunday:
1. Warm up with a brisk walk out to the field to catch horse.
2. Before ride:
All flexibility exercises detailed in Chapter Two – shoulder shrugs, arm circles, side stretches, hip swings and trunk rotation.
2. During ride:
Dismount and walk with horse at least once, aiming to gradually increase effort by including uphill sections to improve aerobic endurance, as well as downhill and rough ground sections.
3. After ride:
All daily stretches as Saturday (Chapter Ten).

Monday:
1. No riding.

3. Cycle to local swimming pool to take part in 'aqua-aerobics' class and then cycle home – a round trip of 10km (six miles) (car permitted when dark and/or wet!).

Tuesday:
1. Morning:
Ride / hack as normal.
2. Afternoon:
Warm up by grooming etc. for at least ten minutes.
All stretching and strengthening exercises detailed in endurance rider exercises (beginning with only ten repetitions of each and gradually building up to twenty when ready).
After exercise – all daily stretches (Chapter Ten).

Wednesday:
As Sunday.

Thursday:
1. Morning:
Ride / hack as normal.
2. Evening:
Long soak in the bath followed by all advanced stretches detailed in Chapter Ten – lying hamstring, adductor, lower back and gluteal, and hip flexor muscles.

Friday:
As Tuesday.

Summary of Rider Fitness Training for Endurance:

• Train for aerobic endurance to increase general fitness and to prevent fatigue on long rides / competitions
• Train for core stability and strength to be able to maintain good posture and a correct, balanced position in the saddle
• Train to improve and maintain flexibility to be able to stay relaxed, comfortable, and effective in the saddle
• Exercise / stretch regularly to become more aware of your own body and muscles – learn to feel how you and your horse are working
• Use flatwork and school sessions as well as hacks to improve general riding skills – trot diagonals, leading legs etc. – and to develop a better understanding of how the horse's muscles work under the rider

• Return to the start position and then repeat the exercise in reverse order by beginning with a twist to the right this time
• Continue to twist and turn until the ball has been placed on the bale ten times in total
• Breathe normally, maintain good posture in your upper body and keep both feet flat on the ground throughout.

Side-step and Squat: to stretch the adductor muscles and strengthen the legs – gluteals, quadriceps, hamstrings and calves (*see* pictures 36a and 36b)

> **Tips:** advance this exercise when ready by balancing without the use of the polo stick.

• Stand on the bale with feet together, use a polo stick (or broom) for balance

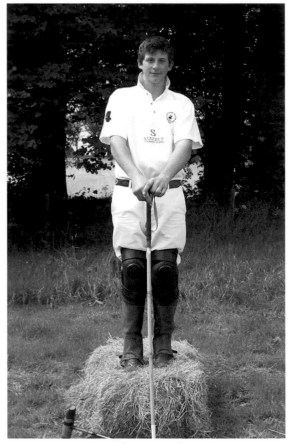 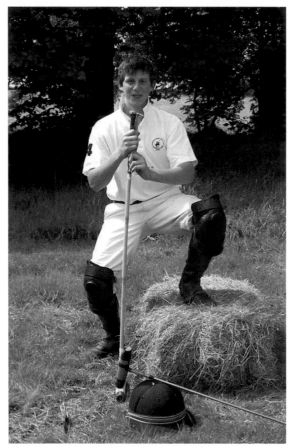

36a Side-step and squat   *36b Step off the bale and squat*

• Step to the side, off the bale, with your right foot and bend both knees to squat down until you feel a stretch on the inside of your left thigh
• Return to the start position, push hard on the ground with your right foot to spring back to the bale
• Step to the side, off the bale, with your left foot to repeat the exercise
• Continue to alternate legs until you have stepped to the side twenty times in total
• Breathe out through your mouth as you squat each time and in through your nose as you spring back to the bale
• Keep good posture, stay relaxed and take your time – avoid using your arms on the stick to assist the return to the bale

Cycle Crunches: to strengthen the abdominal and oblique muscles (*see* pictures 37a and 37b)

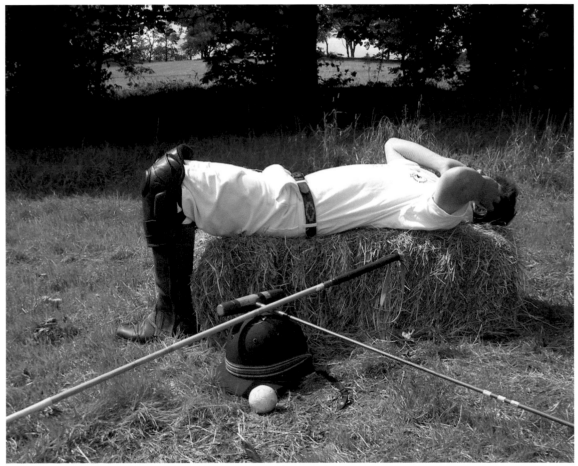

37a Cycle crunches

CHAPTER TEN

INJURY PREVENTION

All athletes, whether equine or human, undoubtedly will suffer an injury or two at some point in their sporting career. We rely on doctors and vets to diagnose, treat and prescribe medication for acute injuries but the aim of this chapter is to look at some of the preventative measures that can be taken to reduce the risks of developing chronic or recurring problems.

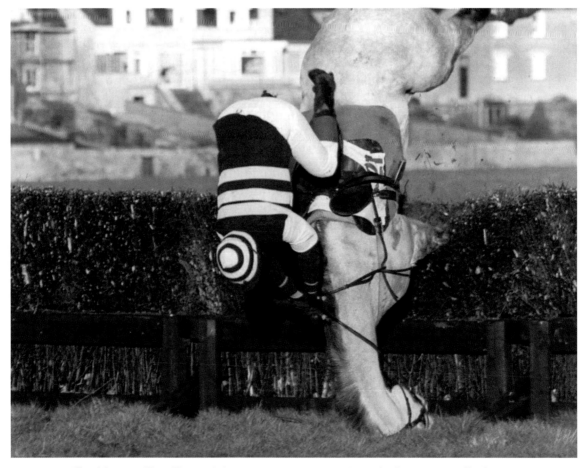

All athletes will suffer an injury or two at some point – both parties walked away!

Two – shoulder shrugs, arm circles, trunk rotation, side stretches and hip swings – are a useful addition to any warm-up routine but listed below are some common yard duties that also provide a practical means of preparing for exercise.

Mucking Out:
Mucking out a straw bed is virtually guaranteed to warm you up. Using a pitch fork, a shovel and a brush will create enough movement in your muscles and joints to raise your body temperature and elevate your heart rate, provided you don't spend too much time just leaning on them! Steady paced mucking out for ten minutes or more should have you feeling warm enough to remove an outer layer of clothing and therefore ready to exercise. Shavings beds and similar types of bedding may not generate the same amount of effort, especially if deep littered, so it could take a little longer to feel warm but several trips to the muck heap with a loaded wheelbarrow should still have the desired effect.

Muck Heap Tidying:
Forking up the edges of the muck heap and then tramping down the contents will help to enhance the rotting process and prevent the muck heap from taking over the entire yard. The effort and the movement required will certainly get you feeling warm enough to exercise.

Yard Sweeping:
Steady, rhythmical sweeping will gradually elevate your heart rate and raise your body temperature. Ten minutes of continuous sweeping should get you feeling warm enough to exercise and it also provides a good opportunity to try using both arms in an effort to combat any one-sidedness in your body. Using your weaker arm will initially feel very awkward but practice will pay off and you will soon reap the rewards of improved muscle balance – and a nice tidy yard!

Grooming:
Thorough grooming will create enough movement in your body to elevate your heart rate and warm up your muscles. However, care must be taken to use the correct practice to gain the most from your grooming session. Use both arms, right arm on the right side of the horse and left arm on the left side, and bend your knees rather than your back, to reach lower areas.

Strapping:
Old-fashioned strapping will help to stimulate muscle contraction in your horse and will also serve as a useful warm-up for your own muscles. Use of both arms is important to maintain balance in your routine but as little

as five minutes of concentrated effort will go a long way towards improving your horse's muscle tone and your own!

Track Raking:
You may be lucky enough to have a mechanised system of caring for your riding school surface but the 'track' area around the edge of the arena is always the area that suffers the most wear and tear. Raking in the displaced surface by hand will certainly warm up your body in preparation for exercise and it will also ensure that your horse continues to enjoy an even working surface which will protect his joints.

Poo Picking:
Pushing a wheelbarrow and walking around the field or the riding arena will get your body working and serve as a useful warm up. Collecting manure regularly will protect your grazing land or riding surface and a little at a time will not only keep you on top of the situation but will also provide an ideal, practical and timesaving warm-up routine.

Warm-Up Before a Competition
The amount of time needed to warm up will vary depending on the circumstances, the weather and the individual.

The Horse:
In the horse's case, part of the warming up process may be just getting used to a new environment if travelling has been involved to compete away from home. A long journey will have affected the horse both physically and mentally so this must be taken into consideration when planning the timetable for the day. New surroundings will generally cause excitement so sufficient settling down time must be allowed before the actual process of warming up can begin. An important part of the warm-up routine is to promote suppleness through relaxation so any tension in the muscles brought about by competition eagerness must be released before progress can be made.

The Rider:
Competition nerves can also affect the rider's ability to concentrate on warming up correctly and there is a real danger of overdoing it in the warm-up arena. How many times have you ridden through the entire test just one more time to make sure? Or gone over those practice fences just a few more times to convince yourself you're ready? Relaxed, supple muscles are just as important in the rider's body if tension is to be avoided in both parties. This can only be achieved by allowing sufficient time to work through a gradual, calm and relevant warm-up routine. Rushing around at

the last minute only adds to the danger of injuries occurring and neither an ill-prepared nor an exhausted horse and rider combination are likely to perform at their best!

The Importance of Cool Down

Vigorous activity will get your heart pounding and your breathing rate elevated to the point of puffing and panting. Thankfully, it's not always necessary to exert yourself to this degree in an exercise session to realise any benefits. However, after exercising it is important to allow your pulse rate and breathing rate to slow down again gradually if they have been elevated above normal levels. It can be very tempting to throw yourself onto the floor in a heap at the end of an exercise session but a more effective means of recovery is to slow the activity gradually so that your pulse and breathing rate begin to slow down while you are still on the move. Cooling down is sometimes known as warming down because the process of allowing your body to recover gradually, whilst continuing to keep your muscles gently on the move, also allows your body temperature to return to normal gradually without the risk of becoming chilled. This helps to prevent the onset of muscular aches and pains often associated with exercise.

The Horse:

At the end of a competition or hard training session, it is more than likely that your horse will be hot, sweaty, and experiencing a high heart and breathing rate. It is already common practice to keep the horse on the move by walking him in hand and allowing him to cool gradually by using a sweat rug of some sort. The amount of time needed to cool down effectively will depend on many factors, including the weather and the degree of stress the horse has suffered, but the gradual cooling process will continue until his vital signs – breathing rate and heart rate – are showing recovery. This means nostrils will no longer be flaring, flanks will no longer be heaving, sweating will slow down or stop, and the pulse rate will drop to near normal. The fitter the horse, the quicker the recovery process will be. More detail on this subject is given in Chapter Eleven – *Training Using A Heart Rate Monitor.*

The Rider:

At the end of your own fitness training session, you may also be feeling hot, sweaty, and experiencing a high heart and breathing rate. Exactly the same principles apply to your own body, as described above for the horse, so a gentle walk around will aid recovery and allow your nostrils to stop flaring, your flanks to stop heaving and your sweating to stop! On cooler days, it may be necessary to put on another layer of clothing to allow you to recover fully without becoming cold. Once your vital signs begin to return to normal, it is worth taking a few moments to work through a simple stretching routine at this point while your muscles are still warm. The fitter you are, the quicker the recovery process will be but a regular stretching programme will help to keep your body supple, less prone to stiffness and better conditioned to cope with the demands of your sport.

Daily Stretches for Riders

The following exercises should be performed on a regular basis, preferably every day, and always when the muscles are warm, so the ideal time to stretch is after an exercise session or after a ride when your muscles will have worked hard and will benefit most from what is known as a maintenance stretching routine. Warm muscles are more pliable and therefore more susceptible to the stretch so a daily routine could also include stretching first thing in the morning when you're nice and warm from your bed or stretching in the evening after a relaxing bath. Cold muscles are less flexible and more likely to become injured if stretched so careful preparation is needed, especially if working outdoors in cold weather. Hold each stretch for fifteen seconds and then repeat after allowing the muscle to relax briefly.

Upper Body Stretches

> **Note:** a guide to the location and function of the muscles can be found at the end of Chapter One.

Triceps (*see* picture 39)
- Hold your arm below the elbow joint
- Aim to ease your elbow towards your head but resist the movement just enough to feel the stretch down the back of your upper arm

Pectorals and Front of Shoulders (*see* picture 40)
- Clasp your hands behind your back
- Ease your hands away from your body by squeezing your shoulder blades together
- Aim to feel the stretch across the top of your chest and shoulders

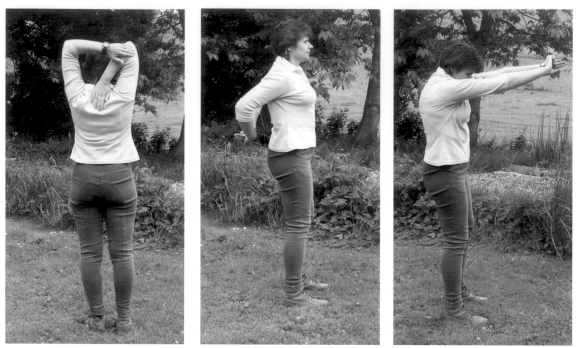

39 Triceps stretch   *40 Pectoral stretch*   *41 Rhomboids stretch*

Rhomboids and Back of Shoulders (*see* picture 41)
- Clasp your hands and hold them out in front of you at shoulder height
- Palms facing outwards, aim to push your hands away from your body until you feel a stretch between your shoulder blades

Lower Body Stretches

Quadriceps (*see* picture 42)
- Lean against something for balance and bend one leg at the knee by catching hold of the ankle
- Bring the heel of that leg towards your bottom until you feel a stretch down the front of the thigh
- Keep your standing leg relaxed at the knee
- Keep both knees together as you stretch and increase the stretch by tilting your pelvis forwards
- Repeat to stretch the other leg

Hamstrings (*see* picture 43)
- Lean on a bent leg with both hands above the knee joint
- Straighten the other leg in front by placing the heel on the ground and sticking your bottom out behind you

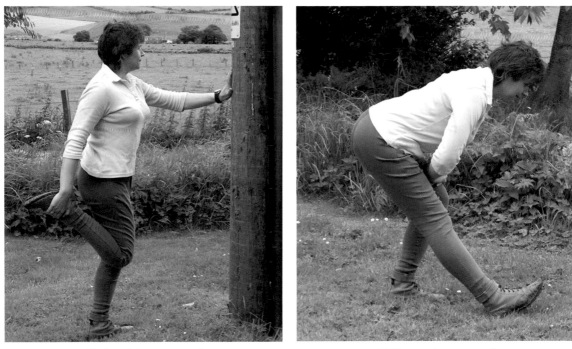

42 Quadriceps stretch   *43 Hamstrings stretch*

• Lower your upper body towards the ground until you feel the stretch down the back of the straight leg – keep the stretching leg locked straight at the knee
• Repeat to stretch the other leg.

Calves (*see* picture 44)
• Lean against a wall (or something secure) and take a step back with one leg
• Keep the heel of your back leg on the ground
• Lean in towards the wall until you feel a stretch in the lower half of your back leg
• Repeat to stretch the other leg
• The stretch can be increased by stepping back further from the wall but remember to keep your heel on the ground

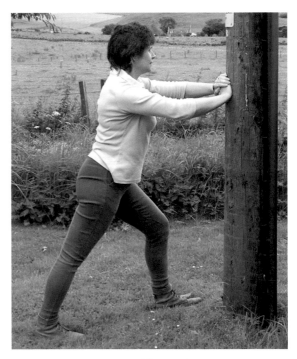

44 Calf stretch

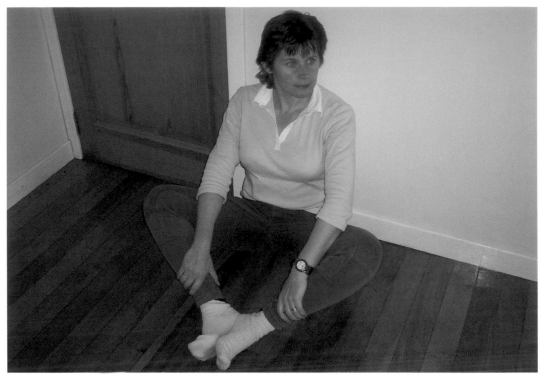

46 Adductor stretch

• Hold the stretch for twenty seconds and then allow the muscles to relax briefly, by straightening your legs, before stretching them again for a further twenty seconds
• As your flexibility increases, you may find you can comfortably progress the stretch by placing your hands on the inside of your knees and applying gentle downward pressure
• Keep good posture in your upper body, stay relaxed and breathe normally

Alternative Adductor Stretch: (*see* picture 47)
• Sit with both legs out in front as shown – it is important to remain comfortable so this will dictate the angle of your legs!
• Keeping both legs flat to the floor, begin to move your hands forward along the floor until you feel the stretch on the inside of both thighs
• Hold this position for twenty seconds and then relax the muscles briefly, by sitting up, before repeating the stretch for a further twenty seconds
• Keep good posture in your upper body, reach forwards by folding from your hips, stay relaxed and breathe normally

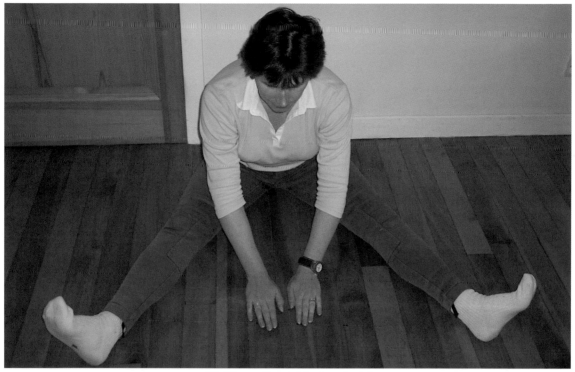

47 Alternative adductor stretch

• As your flexibility improves, you will find that you can reach further along the floor with each stretch – widening the angle of your legs will also intensify the stretch

Lower Back and Gluteal Muscles

To be able to move with the horse, the rider must have relaxed, flexible muscles in the lumbar region. Many people suffer from lower back pain at some point in their lives and this can often be the result of poor posture brought about by weak or inflexible muscles. A sedentary lifestyle may cause a general rounding of the back and shoulders which can mean that an effective riding position, balanced and with good posture, becomes difficult to achieve and then to maintain. Back pain can also be the result of poor practice when lifting etc. so it is extremely important to promote symmetry, strength and suppleness in this area to prevent a muscle imbalance developing.

Lower back and gluteal stretch: (*see* pictures 48a and 48b)
• Lie back on the floor and hug both legs with knees bent in towards your chest

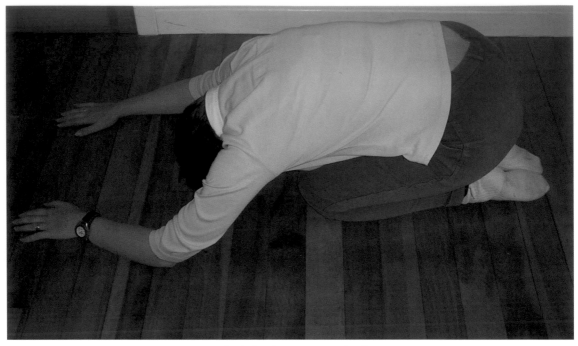

49b Sit back on to your heels

- Tuck your chin in towards your chest and take a deep breath in as you arch your back up towards the sky
- Breathe out again as you relax by sitting back onto your heels while keeping your arms stretched out in front
- Hold this position for fifteen seconds, breathe normally and feel the stretch across your back and shoulders as you aim to increase it by creeping your fingertips across the floor away from your body while keeping your bottom on your heels
- Repeat the whole exercise twice more

Hip Flexor Muscles

As with the hamstring muscles, the hip flexors remain relaxed when in a riding position, or sitting position in general, so they are also prone to adaptive shortening. This can lead to a muscle imbalance and postural problems that will have a direct impact on the rider's effectiveness in the saddle. To prevent this, and to reduce the consequent risk of injury, it is necessary to promote greater flexibility in this muscle group with specific stretches.

Hip Flexor Stretch: (*see* picture 50)
- Position yourself as shown with one leg out in front for balance and the

other leg behind you ready to stretch – lean against a wall or use a broom to aid balance if needed
• Keep the knee of your front leg behind the line of your toe to avoid placing stress on the joint
• Position your other knee sufficiently far enough behind you to feel the stretch down the front of your thigh and the front of your hip – hold for twenty seconds
• Transfer your weight slightly onto your front foot to increase the stretch but maintain good (upright) posture in your upper body
• Relax the muscles briefly after twenty seconds and then repeat the stretch for a further twenty seconds
• Change position to repeat the whole exercise and to stretch the other leg
• Stay relaxed, maintain correct posture and breathe normally
• As your flexibility improves, you may need to position your knee further behind you to develop a greater stretch

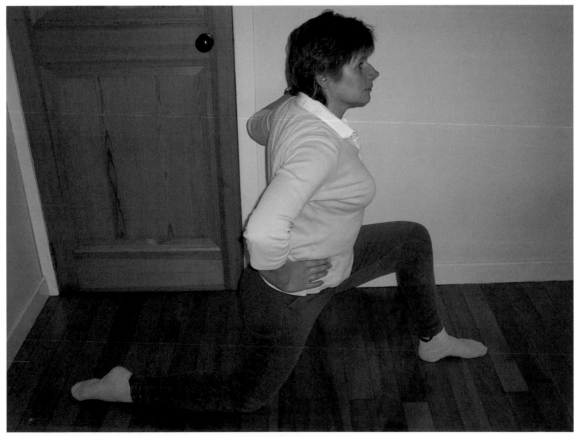

50 Hip flexor stretch

CHAPTER ELEVEN

ONWARDS AND UPWARDS

This chapter is aimed at those who have already established a good level of fitness or those of you who have dutifully followed the programmes detailed in the preceding chapters and now wish to go further.

Riding as a sport can be very time-consuming and those who own horses know all too well just how much time and effort goes into looking after them. Finding spare time to devote to exercise sessions or other non-horsey activities can be virtually impossible but it's important to remember the value of maintaining, at the very least, a good base level of fitness. Consider the fact that in the time it takes to boil the kettle and make a cup of tea you can complete a daily stretching routine! Equal priority should be given to the fitness training of both horse and rider so if you are preparing your horse for more physically demanding challenges then you must also prepare your own body. Time devoted to promoting your own fitness should never be considered a luxury but as an essential in the process of creating a successful partnership between horse and rider.

Keeping all exercise sessions as relevant and sport specific as possible will help to make the best use of time. A rugby player must devote training time to developing the skills needed in his sport but he has no need to embark on the type of fitness training a long-distance runner might employ. Similarly, a horse rider will benefit most from concentrating on functional fitness and therefore has no need to acquire the strength of Arnold Schwarzenegger or the speed of Linford Christie!

The most important elements of any fitness training programme, whether for the horse or the rider, are to take the time to train progressively and to train the body appropriately for the specific demands that will be placed upon it. This requires a structured, planned approach and a regular routine to take you safely and effectively from your current level of fitness through to your 'goal' level.

Goals provide motivation and focus. They could also be called targets, aims or objectives and can be described as long-term or short-term. When planning a training programme, having a number of short-term goals in place will ensure that a sensible time frame can be scheduled to lead to the

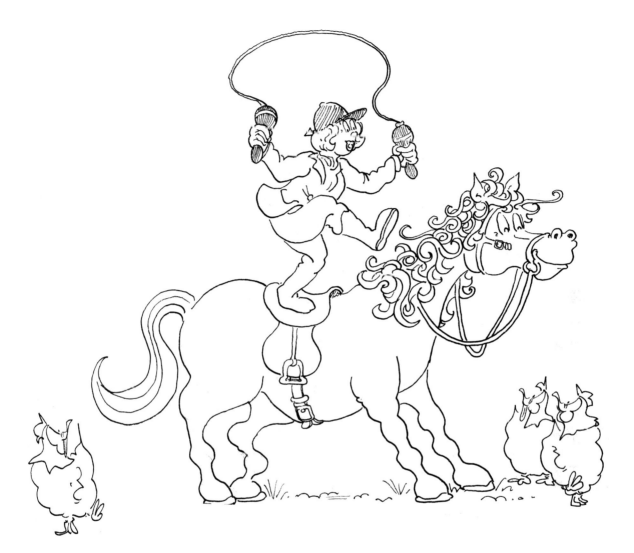

eventual long-term goal. For example, in Chapter Seven the long-term goal is to be able to jog for four kilometres (two and a half miles) so the first short-term goal is to complete the six-week base fitness training programme; the second short-term goal is to complete the next six-week programme leading to ten minutes of continuous jogging; and the third is to add a further two minutes of jogging each week until the long-term goal is reached. Breaking the ultimate goal down in this way, into smaller achievable targets, makes certain that progress continues to be made and that motivation remains high.

Smart Goals

All goals, whether long-term or short-term, must be SMART goals:

S   SPECIFIC

Goals should be as specific to the training programme and / or each exercise session as possible. For example, a goal at the start of a session could be:

Specific – complete ten repetitions of all the flexibility exercises detailed in Chapter Two.

Non specific – do some flexibility exercises.
Vague signposts generally lead to getting lost!

M   MEASURABLE

Measuring improvement can provide great motivation and without such measurements it becomes difficult to monitor progress and chart success.

A   ACHIEVABLE

Goals must be realistic to be achievable. Setting too difficult a goal tends to lead to a feeling of failure and a loss of confidence or interest.

R   RECORDED

Recording progress (test results) provides valuable feedback to help maintain motivation. Writing down goals also increases commitment and helps to keep training on track.

T   TIME PHASED

A training programme must be planned in steps with each step including a short-term goal to be achieved within a specified time frame. Without a time-phased approach there is a tendency to drift along aimlessly and the long-term goal may never be reached.

Taking part in other sports and activities need not detract from the goal of improving fitness for riding. Many relevant skills can be learned and practised without the need to be in the saddle and taking part in other sports will also add interest and variety to any training programme. Known as cross-training, the latter part of this chapter takes a look at some other popular activities that may provide useful additional or alternative fitness training to complement your existing programme. Further progress can also be made by introducing the use of a heart rate monitor to add a more scientific approach. The use of this technology is already widespread in other sports and heart rate monitors are commonly used in endurance riding to ensure that the horses are always fit to continue at each stage. Once the domain of scientists or medical professionals only, heart rate monitors are now relatively inexpensive and widely available to all of us in many forms.

Training Using a Heart Rate Monitor (HRM)

There's a lot to be said in defence of training a horse through 'feel' and many equine experts rely entirely on instinct and their natural 'eye' for a horse to produce fit, well-conditioned animals. The same can be said for many human athletes and their coaches who depend on trusted, tried and tested training methods along with countless years of experience to get results. However, an HRM provides an effective tool to enable the user, at any level, to make the most efficient use of training time by ensuring that all exercises are performed at the appropriate intensity to achieve the desired results. This is particularly useful when training an equine athlete as they are unable to tell the trainer how they are feeling. A human athlete can, of course, let the coach know how they are coping at any stage throughout a training exercise and adjustments can be made to maintain the optimum degree of effort.

HRMs range from simple devices that display only the current heart rate, through to highly complex pieces of equipment that display and record vast amounts of information which can then be downloaded onto a computer and analysed. In all cases, the athlete, equine and human alike, wears a chest (or girth) strap known as a transmitter belt. This picks up the heartbeat and transmits the information to a wristwatch which can be worn by the rider or the trainer on the ground. A constant display on the watch screen shows the current number of heartbeats per minute so any changes in heart rate can be seen the instant they happen.

> **Note:** details of HRM manufacturers can be found in Useful Contacts at the back of this book.

The Horse:
A horse's resting heart rate (RHR) gives a clear indication of its general state of health. It is important to measure the heart rate at rest, when the horse is in a relaxed and familiar situation, as any unusual or strange activity will

cause excitement resulting in an increase in the heart rate. The measurement can be taken manually by locating a pulse or, more accurately, by using a HRM – The Polar® VetCheck is a useful product as it is hand-held and easier to use without disturbing the horse. An adult horse's RHR is usually in the range of 25 to 40 beats per minute (bpm) but sudden excitement, fear or anticipation of exercise can cause a rapid rise to over 100 bpm so it's advisable to record the heart rate over a period of several days to establish a benchmark measurement. If the RHR is 6 bpm higher than normal, the horse is undergoing some form of stress. This could be an indication of an impending infection or an injury that is not yet apparent but it could also be the result of a hard training session the previous day from which the horse has not yet fully recovered. This elevation in RHR would alert the owner to a potential problem and a further investigation into the cause at this stage might prevent a minor health issue becoming a serious one.

The recovery heart rate is another indicator of the horse's state of health. Monitoring the heart rate at the end of an exercise session provides a clear indication of the degree of stress and strain the horse has undergone and the current fitness level. The most significant drop in heart rate should occur within the first sixty to ninety seconds after exercise and a near normal (pre-exercise) heart rate should be achieved within ten minutes of recovery time at the end of the session. If the heart rate fails to drop significantly in this time, or after thirty minutes at the most, it indicates the horse is under intense physical stress and may be suffering from pain or the symptoms of over-training. Clearly, action must be taken to alleviate the stress and steps taken to identify the cause which may mean reassessing the horse's training programme.

The following reliable recovery rate values have been established for use by vets at endurance event checkpoints to ensure that all horses remain fit to continue:

1 Fit to continue – a heart rate of less than 68 bpm after ten minutes of recovery.
2 Check up required – a heart rate above 68 bpm after ten minutes of recovery time requires a further check within an additional twenty minute recovery period.
3 Not permitted to continue – a heart rate above 68 bpm after the total thirty minute recovery period shows the horse to be unfit to continue and is a cause for concern.

A heart rate monitor also provides a means of monitoring the horse's progress during a fitness training programme. Various fitness tests can be used to establish the current fitness level and to check that the horse is adapting appropriately to the prescribed programme. However, fitness test results can only be used for comparison purposes if the same protocol has been followed each time. Known as standardisation, this means that an identical procedure is needed in everything from the activities of the previous day through to the warm-up method used on the day, feeding times and the time of day the test is performed. When interpreting results, slight changes in the test situation such as weather, temperature and ground conditions should all be recorded and taken into consideration. Unless you have access to indoor facilities such as an equine treadmill it can be difficult to achieve this level of standardisation but it is still possible to accumulate enough useful information to provide an insight into how the horse is responding to training.

Provided an appropriate period of progressive training time has been allowed, success will be shown in the fitness test results in one of two ways:

1. The horse is able to complete the same task at the same speed as before but with a lower heart rate than before which indicates increased fitness.

2. The horse is able to complete longer tasks at greater speeds but with the same heart rate as before (no higher) which indicates increased fitness.

The Cardiac Recovery Index or CRI-Test is often used by vets when evaluating a horse's fitness. A combination of both rest and recovery heart rate is used and the test is normally taken after the horse has been exercised and then allowed ten minutes of recovery time.

CRI-Test Protocol

1 Choose a flat area to create an 80 metre out and back course – 40 metres out and 40 metres back.

2 Measure the horse's heart rate (basic heart rate) at the end of the ten minute recovery period after exercise.

3 Trot the horse, in hand, around the 80 metre course – begin timing the horse at the start of the trot.

4 Exactly one minute after the start of the trot measure the horse's heart rate again – the trot is likely to take between 25 and 30 seconds so the horse will have the remaining time as recovery before the heart rate is taken.

CRI-Test Protocol (continued)

5 The horse should be observed carefully during the trot for any signs of lameness or discomfort.

6 The second heart rate measurement must always be taken exactly one minute after the first to compensate for differences in speed. Fast-trotting horses have a longer recovery period than the slower ones.

7 According to an established criterion concerning a horse's fitness, the recovery heart rate (second measurement) should be two to three beats below the basic heart rate (first measurement) to be considered fit to pass.

8 If the horse fails the CRI-Test (heart rate fails to drop) a further recovery period is allowed before the heart rate is taken again. If after thirty minutes (from the start of the trot) the horse is still unable to pass, it would be considered unfit to continue with any exercise and would need careful observation.

All horses are individuals so variations will be seen across the board in terms of resting heart rate, breathing rate and body temperature. It is therefore very important to know your horse well and to have a record (compiled over a suitable period of time) of all 'normal' readings in each case. By recording the results of fitness tests throughout the horse's training, a more precise map of progress can be drawn and all training sessions can be kept appropriate to the needs of each individual animal. Not all horses will respond in the same way to the same training programme. Whatever your ultimate goal, whether that be increased speed, increased strength or increased stamina, the use of an equine heart rate monitor takes all guesswork out of the equation and ensures that the horse continues to train at the appropriate effort level and intensity to achieve the desired results.

The Rider:
One big difference between training yourself and training your horse is that you always know exactly how hard you are working – so you also know when you're slacking! Every exercise you do creates an instant response in your body making it easy to feel whether you've targeted the desired muscle group and achieved the correct level of intensity. However, as

explained earlier in the book, your body adapts quickly to progressive training so exercises that initially feel challenging soon become much more manageable. To ensure continuing progress, and also to make the best use of available training time, the use of a HRM helps each individual to exercise at an appropriate effort level to stimulate the desired response.

The first step is to measure and record your resting heart rate (RHR). Ideally, this should be done first thing in the morning before you even get out of bed but, as this is not always practical, it should be taken when you are at rest or in a relaxed state. Take a reading, always at the same time of day and in the same circumstances, over a period of several days and then use the average figure as your actual resting heart rate. The average adult RHR in Britain is between 70 and 75 beats per minute (bpm) but many individual variations occur as this is largely an hereditary factor. Just because someone has a lower RHR than you does not necessarily mean they are fitter than you! Whatever your current rate is, as you become fitter your RHR becomes lower. This is because your heart becomes stronger and more efficient meaning it can pump out a larger volume of oxygenated blood to fuel the working muscles with each single beat. (It is worth noting that tests show this rule not to apply to horses.)

The next step is to discover your maximum heart rate (MHR). To find your true maximum you would need to push your body through intense exercise until you dropped – quite literally! Obviously, this is not a popular option so various sub-maximal tests have been designed to allow an educated prediction to be made. These fitness tests are readily available at most gyms or fitness centres and are not at all strenuous so they provide a much more appealing option. However, the simplest method of predicting your MHR is to use an existing formula. The formula considers the maximum human heart rate to be 220 bpm (the foetal heart rate?) and then for each year of your life you subtract 1 bpm. For example, a 40-year-old adult would have a predicted MHR of 180 bpm (220 bpm — 40 years = 180 bpm). This is by no means an exact science but the results will provide a sensible benchmark figure from which to begin.

By using a heart rate monitor as you exercise, it becomes possible to ensure that each session is being performed at the correct intensity to achieve the desired results. This is done by taking a percentage of your MHR, depending on your goal, to calculate your target heart rate zone (THRZ). As our goal is to continue improving your fitness for riding and to build on the aerobic endurance already achieved, the most effective THRZ is between 75% and 85% of your MHR. For example, a 40-year-old rider with a predicted MHR of 180 bpm would need to exercise within the range of 135 bpm and 153 bpm (180 x 75% = 135 and 180 x 85% = 153) to make the most of all aerobic endurance training sessions. No wasted training time and no slacking!

These measurements could all be taken manually by locating your pulse and counting the number of beats per minute at each stage in the session but this would involve slowing down or stopping. Exercise will, of course, elevate your heart rate but as you become fitter your heart rate will decrease faster when you stop (quicker recovery) therefore making it difficult to achieve accurate readings when counting beats in this way. A heart rate monitor provides instant information allowing you to stay on the move (no slacking again!) and the constant display makes working within the optimal THRZ very simple.

Cross-Training for Fitness

The most effective way to become fitter for any sport is to take part in that sport. Therefore, the best way to improve fitness for riding is to ride!   This is true but not always practical as not all riders own horses and not all horse owners use their riding time to improve their own fitness. Most riders, whether horse owners or not, will admit to concentrating far more on what their horse is doing while they are in the saddle than on themselves. All the exercises detailed in this book are designed to be performed unmounted for that very reason. Fitness and flexibility for riding can only be improved by training the muscles of the body to cope with the stresses that riding will place upon them. This type of training requires correct technique at all times to be effective so by removing the horse from the equation, the rider has total control over the movements required to perform each exercise correctly and, after all, practice makes perfect.

Many other activities involve exercises and movements which can be of benefit to the rider wishing to become fitter for riding without the need to be in the saddle. This can be particularly useful for weekly or infrequent riders or even for those times when weather, ground conditions or lameness might disrupt your normal riding schedule. Listed below are some activities that complement riding well by utilising similar muscle groups and promoting useful skills:

Yoga:
- Promotes body awareness
- Teaches breathing and relaxation techniques
- Increases flexibility
  Contact: The British Wheel Of Yoga – http://www.bwy.org.uk

Pilates:
- Promotes body awareness
- Teaches breathing, balance and coordination techniques

- Increases core strength and stability
  Contact: The Pilates Foundation (UK) – http://www.pilatesfoundation.com

Swimming:
- Non weight-bearing aerobic exercise (less stressful on the body than jogging)
- Teaches correct breathing techniques
- Promotes joint mobility (varies depending on stroke used)
  Contact: Swimming Pools UK – http://www.local.co.uk/uk/swimming_pools

Cycling:
- Aerobic (heart and lung) training exercise
- Promotes balance
- Increases muscle endurance
  Contact: British Cycling – http://www.britishcycling.org.uk

Rollerblading / Skating / Cross-Country Skiing:
- Aerobic exercise
- Teaches rhythm and pace control
- Improves coordination and symmetry
  Contact: http://www.mindbodysoul.gov.uk
          http://www.iceskating.org.uk
          English Ski Council – http://www.escnordic.org.uk

Martial Arts:
- Enhances natural reflexes
- Increases mental focus
- Promotes mobility and flexibility
  Contact: Martial Arts Clubs (UK) – http://www.martialartsclubs.com

Judo:
- Teaches balance, coordination and control of body movements
- Promotes mobility and flexibility
- Teaches how to roll on landing – a useful skill in the event of a fall!
  Contact: British Judo Association – http://www.britishjudo.org.uk

Dance Classes:
- Aerobic exercise (depending on type of dance)
- Promotes coordination
- Teaches correct posture / graceful movement!
  Contact: http://www.danceweb.co.uk

Other sports can also provide useful aerobic endurance training such as tennis, squash, badminton etc. but as they use one side of your body more than the other, they are less useful in terms of developing greater symmetry and balance across your body for riding. However, to improve fitness in general, any activity is better than no activity at all!

CHAPTER TWELVE

PERSONALISE
YOUR PROGRAMME

Many of the exercises detailed in this book are relevant to more than one specific discipline. For example, in Chapter Seven the 'jack knives' exercise is used to strengthen the abdominal muscles and in Chapter Nine the 'cycle crunches' exercise also serves the same purpose so these two exercises are actually interchangeable. As highlighted earlier, your body adapts quickly to a progressive training programme so a plateau may eventually be reached in some areas of your exercise routine. Exchanging one exercise for another ensures that progress continues to be made in such cases as using different exercises to target the same muscle group provides an excellent way of keeping your body working and adds variety to your routine. However, it is always advisable to practise each individual exercise enough times to allow your muscles an opportunity to learn the pattern of movement required, before asking them to perform a new movement. Listed below are the main muscle groups targeted in Section Two – *Sport Specific Fitness Training –*

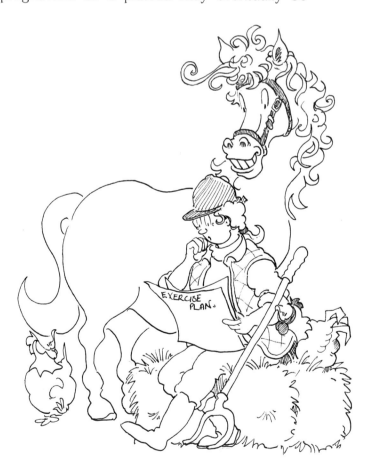

and a guide to locating a variety of exercises aimed at each group which are all interchangeable:

Trunk / Core Stability Muscles:
- A leg at each corner – Chapter Four
- Bucking bronco – Chapter Four
- The plank – Chapter Five
- Superman plank – Chapter Eight

Abdominals:
- Tummy tucks – Chapter Six
- Jack knives – Chapter Seven
- Girth tightener – Chapter Eight
- Cycle crunches – Chapter Nine

Quadriceps (and other leg muscles):
- Travelling front lunges – Chapter Five
- Front lunges – Chapter Six
- Step ups – Chapter Seven
- Leg ups – Chapter Eight

Adductors (and other leg muscles):
- Fat horse squats – Chapter Four
- Travelling wide squats – Chapter Five
- Forward seat squats – Chapter Six
- Side step and squat – Chapter Nine

Heart And Lungs:
- Heel kicks / knee lifts (jog) – Chapter Five
- Side shuttles – Chapter Six
- Hop overs – Chapter Eight
- Twister – Chapter Eight

Putting It All Together

Earlier in this book I suggested that each rider should aim to exercise (off the horse) for at least one hour each week. The following routines show how this can be done in a variety of ways to make it easy to fit your exercise sessions into your existing routine. Using a mixture of exercises from different disciplines helps to add interest and there is no reason why an event rider should not take part in the polo player's routine!

Three sessions each week – twenty minutes each session:

Monday
- Ten minutes – warm up with a brisk walk or jog
- Eight minutes – all rider exercises detailed in Chapter Eight – leg ups / hop overs / girth tightener / superman plank (or plank) / twister
- Two minutes – all daily stretches detailed in Chapter Ten – lower body / upper body

Wednesday
- Ten minutes – warm up with a brisk walk or jog
- Eight minutes – all rider exercises detailed in Chapter Four – a leg at each corner / bucking bronco / fat horse squats / heels down
- Two minutes – all daily stretches detailed in Chapter Ten – lower body / upper body

Friday
- Ten minutes – warm up with a brisk walk or jog
- Ten minutes – all advanced stretches detailed in Chapter Ten – lying hamstring stretch / adductor stretch / lower back and gluteal stretch / hip flexor stretch

Four sessions each week – fifteen minutes each session:

Monday
- Five minutes – warm up with a brisk walk or jog
- Eight minutes – all flexibility exercises detailed in Chapter Two – shoulder shrugs / arm circles / side stretches / hip swings / trunk rotation
- Two minutes – all daily stretches detailed in Chapter Ten – lower body / upper body

Tuesday
- Twelve minutes – Preliminary Drill One detailed in Chapter Five
- Three minutes – the plank exercise detailed in Chapter Five plus all daily stretches detailed in Chapter Ten – lower body / upper body

Thursday
- Three minutes – warm up with brisk walk or alternative activity
- Ten minutes – Jumping Circuit detailed in Chapter Six
- Two minutes – all daily stretches detailed in Chapter Ten – lower body / upper body

Saturday
- Five minutes – warm up with brisk walk or jog
- Ten minutes – all advanced stretches detailed in Chapter Ten – lying hamstring / adductor / lower back and gluteal / hip flexor muscles

Six sessions each week – ten minutes each session:

Tuesday
- Ten minutes – power walk or jog plus daily leg stretches detailed in Chapter Ten

Wednesday
- Five minutes – warm up with brisk walk, jog, or alternative activity
- Five minutes – all daily joint mobility exercises detailed in Chapter Four – neck / elbows / wrists / trunk and spine / hips and pelvis / knees / ankles

Thursday
- Ten minutes – power walk or jog plus leg stretches (as Tuesday)

Friday
- Five minutes – warm up with brisk walk, jog, or alternative activity
- Five minutes – selected flexibility exercises from Chapter Two – side stretches / hip swings / trunk rotation plus all daily stretches detailed in Chapter Ten – lower body / upper body

Saturday
- Ten minutes – power walk or jog plus leg stretches (as Thursday)

Sunday
- Ten minutes – all advanced stretches detailed in Chapter Ten – lying hamstring / adductor / lower back and gluteal / hip flexor muscles

---

Note: make sure your muscles are warm before starting to stretch.

Update Your Training Record

In Chapter One, the Merrell® Ten Minute Challenge was introduced as a way of assessing your aerobic fitness, and the Sit And Reach Test as a guide to your lower back and hamstring muscle flexibility. Planning to repeat these tests after a period of training (minimum of six weeks) can provide an extra bit of motivation to keep you going on the days when you are feeling a bit lazy! The results can be used as a comparison to chart your progress, to provide an incentive and also to highlight any areas of your training that may need greater attention. Depending on your original results, the aim of your training programme is either to improve on the original score or to maintain the level previously achieved so an update will provide all the necessary information.

The Merrell® Ten Minute Challenge:

The time taken to complete the 800 metre (half-mile) walk test will decrease as you become fitter and you may wish to progress to another form of aerobic endurance testing which involves running in place of walking. As with the walking test, the running test involves timing yourself over a set distance and this test uses 2400 metres (one and a half miles). You could create a running track around the edge of your riding arena but you would need to run twenty complete laps (40 metres by 20 metres) to reach your target. This could prove to be quite boring so an alternative plan is to measure a suitable area of road or track in your car instead. Due to the distance involved, this test is not suitable for anyone new to running and should only be taken by those who have previous experience or have built up their running ability gradually by following the progressive programme in Chapter Three. Compare your time in minutes and seconds against the following chart which is broken down into age groups and is specific to either male or female participants.

Note: always warm up thoroughly before beginning this test.

Source: The Institute For Aerobics Research (1994).

The One And A Half Mile Running Test For Aerobic Fitness

Age	20 - 29	30 - 39	40 - 49	50 - 59	60 +
Women					
High	< 12:50	< 13:42	< 14:30	< 15:56	< 16:19
Above average	12:51-14:23	13:43-15:07	14:31-15:56	15:57-16:57	16:20-17:45
Average	14:24-15:26	15:08-15:57	15:57-16:58	16:58-17:55	17:46-18:44
Below average	15:27-16:33	15:58-17:14	16:59-18:00	17:56-18:49	18:45-19:21
Low	> 16:34	> 17:15	> 18:01	> 18:50	> 19:22
Men					
High	< 10:15	< 10:46	< 11:43	< 12:50	< 13:52
Above average	10:16-11:40	10:47-12:19	11:44-13:13	12:51-14:23	13:53-15:28
Average	11:41-12:51	12:20-13:36	13:14-14:29	14:24-15:26	15:29-16:43
Below average	12:52-14:13	13:37-14:52	14:30-15:41	15:27-16:43	16:44-18:00
Low	> 14:14	> 14:53	> 15:42	> 16:44	> 18:01

Sit and Reach Test:

If you previously scored well on this test for lower back and hamstring muscle flexibility, then your aim must be to maintain that degree of flexibility throughout your life. Tight hamstring muscles, along with weak abdominal muscles, are known to contribute to lower back pain so this is an area of particular concern for all riders. The daily stretches and advanced stretches detailed in Chapter Ten ensure that all the muscle groups most affected by the sport of riding are kept in good condition and that existing flexibility is maintained. Continuing to follow a regular stretching routine will also help to improve flexibility and any progress made will be shown by an improved score on the Sit And Reach Test.

Body Composition Testing:

Not all riders choose to take part in competitive equestrian sports but as you progress in your riding your body composition becomes an area of greater importance. To be fit for life, as well as fit for riding, it is important to keep your body composition – muscle versus fat – within an acceptable and healthy ratio. The most accurate method of determining your body fat involves being totally submerged in water so this is obviously not a practical or popular method for most! Various other simpler methods exist and most gyms and leisure centres have the equipment needed to do a test for you. Some weighing scales for home use also have a facility for measuring body fat but it's important to note that the results produced by any of these methods, whether using gym or home equipment, are not an exact science and therefore can't be considered entirely accurate. However, if the same method is used each time, then the results are still useful in terms of indicating progress.

The Body Mass Index (BMI) is another method of predicting fat mass which is often used by doctors, although this is now becoming less common as the results are often very misleading. Your BMI is calculated by dividing your weight in kilograms by the square of your height in metres. Unfortunately, this formula does not take into consideration the fact that muscle mass weighs heavier than fat mass so a fit, lean, muscular person could produce a BMI result which would place them in an unhealthy, overweight or obese body composition range and would clearly be incorrect. For example, the rugby player Jonny Wilkinson is well known to most. He measures 1.75 metres and weighs 85 kgs giving him a BMI of 27.7. The acceptable, healthy range on the BMI scale for adult men is between 20 and 25 so the formula places Jonny Wilkinson in the unhealthy and, in fact, obese category for his height. This is clearly not an accurate result as the naked eye can see that his body weight is the result of muscle mass and not fat.

The simplest, most useful method of measuring your body composition, in terms of assessing your health, is to use circumferential measurements.

Put simply, a pear-shaped body is healthier than an apple-shaped body so your waist measurement should be smaller than your hip measurement. The waist to hip ratio provides a means of predicting each individual's level of risk in terms of weight related illness such as heart disease, diabetes and high blood-pressure. To calculate your waist to hip ratio simply divide your waist measurement by your hip measurement e.g. waist of 66 cms (26 inches) and hips of 91 cms (36 inches) = 0.72 (66 divided by 91 or 26 divided by 36 = 0.72) and then compare your final figure with the following chart which is broken down into age groups and genders.

Body Composition – Waist To Hip Ratio

Age	20 - 29	30 - 39	40 - 49	50 - 59	60 +
Women					
Low risk	< 0.71	< 0.73	< 0.74	< 0.75	< 0.77
Moderate risk	0.71 - 0.78	0.73 - 0.79	0.74 - 0.80	0.75 - 0.81	0.77 - 0.83
High risk	0.78 - 0.81	0.79 - 0.84	0.80 - 0.86	0.81 - 0.88	0.83 - 0.90
Very high risk	> 0.81	> 0.84	> 0.86	> 0.88	> 0.90
Men					
Low risk	< 0.82	< 0.83	< 0.86	< 0.87	< 0.88
Moderate risk	0.82 - 0.87	0.83 - 0.91	0.86 - 0.92	0.87 - 0.94	0.88 - 0.95
High risk	0.87 - 0.94	0.91 - 0.95	0.92 - 1.0	0.94 - 1.01	0.95 - 1.02
Very high risk	> 0.94	> 0.95	> 1.0	> 1.01	> 1.02

Excessive body weight created by stored fat is both unhealthy and undesirable. Apart from the aforementioned health concerns, it also restricts the range of movement around joints and will make the rider much less effective in the saddle. As the subject of this book is fitness for riding, it is important to stress that some body fat is essential to health so it is possible to have too little as well as too much. A healthy, balanced diet coupled with a sensible, progressive programme of exercise is the most effective way to reduce, and then maintain, weight and body fat safely. There is no such thing as a 'quick fix' and crash diets simply don't work. A thin horse with visible ribs, dull coat and a noticeable lack of energy would not be considered healthy or fit for exercise so an excessively thin person is not necessarily a fit or healthy person either!

Opposite: Demonstrating the flexibility required for Le Trec

FOOD AND FUN TO FUEL FITNESS TRAINING

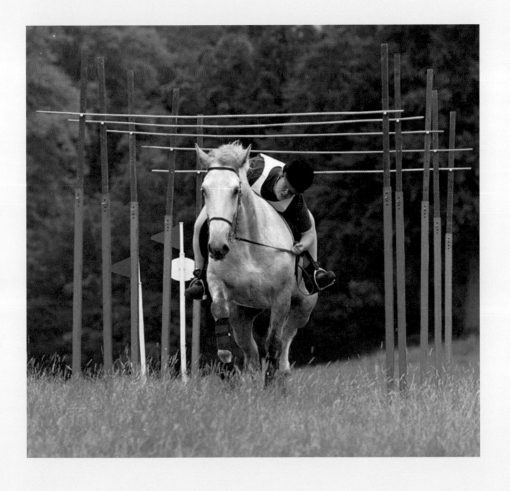

CHAPTER THIRTEEN

DO YOU EAT LIKE A HORSE?

The subject of food and nutrition for both equines and humans is an enormous one, but how many horse riders pay as much attention to their own diet as they do their horse's? It is beyond the scope of this book to advise on feeding programmes for horses but applying the same principles used when feeding horses to our own eating habits could prove to be of enormous benefit to today's busy horse owner. In fact, being accused of eating like a horse is actually something to be proud of!

It's all too common to see riders down at the stables grabbing a bar of chocolate to keep them going before they ride as they have rushed to the yard straight from work and won't be eating properly until they go home – if at all. Sadly, those same riders tend to complain about a constant feeling of tiredness and generally suffer more than their fair share of illnesses throughout the year. Eating a balanced diet is the only way to improve this situation and the best source of tips for healthier eating may actually come straight from the horse's mouth.

One of the first things any student of horsemanship learns is the list of information known as 'The Rules Of Feeding'. There is no question over the importance of these rules and they have certainly stood the test of time by being passed down through the generations.

Here is a reminder:

1. Feed little and often
2. Feed plenty of bulk
3. Feed according to age, size and work being done
4. Make no sudden changes to diet or routine
5. Keep to the same daily feeding hours
6. Feed only good quality, clean forage
7. Feed succulents daily
8. Allow at least one hour after feeding before exercising
9. Water before feeding

Feed little and often:

Horses in the wild are grazing animals so by nature they would continue to eat a little at a time throughout the entire day. Their main form of defence from predators would be to take 'flight' so for this reason horses have small stomachs designed to hold only small amounts at any one time. It is important to imitate this when feeding a stabled horse by providing their daily rations in smaller amounts spread over the day.

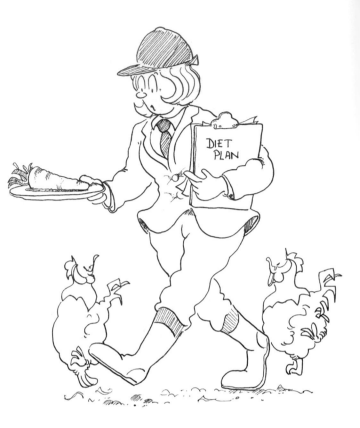

What can *we* learn from this?

Our own ancestors were 'hunter gatherers' and would walk great distances in search of food – much further than your out of town supermarket! They would use nuts and berries to keep up their energy levels throughout the day and eating was purely for survival, unlike today when we treat ourselves to something nice and generally totally unnecessary on a regular basis.

Most of us find it difficult to eat 'three square meals' a day and long gaps will often be left between meals causing a drop in blood sugar levels and, consequently, a drop in energy. By eating a balanced diet split into four or five smaller meals spread over the day we could make sure that we get enough calories to fuel our daily activities without experiencing those 'lows' that make us reach for the chocolate bars.

Feed plenty of bulk:

Bulk is provided by grass or, in the case of the stabled horse, replaced by hay or similar. Plenty of bulk is needed to ensure that the digestive organs are kept filled and working, as without adequate supplies the digestive process is unable to function as nature intended.

What can *we* learn from this?

Our own bodies also need 'bulk' in the form of fibre to ensure our own digestive system is kept in good working order. Good sources of fibre can be found in wholemeal foods, whole grain cereals, and most fruits and vegetables, especially if you leave the skins on. Fibre is also thought to help reduce cholesterol levels and by aiding the passage of foods through the system it helps to prevent diseases of the bowel.

Feed according to the work being done:

If the training load increases so must the amount of food. If the training becomes lighter then the amount of food needed must also decrease. The ratio of concentrated food to bulk will also vary depending on the work-load but, as a general rule, if concentrates go up then bulk goes down and vice versa. A larger horse will need a larger total daily intake of food than a smaller horse – simple!

What can *we* learn from this?

It really *is* that simple! Eat what is required to fuel your daily activities and no more. If you want to lose weight it becomes a simple case of calories in, versus calories out. However, it's not all about losing weight as we need to eat the right mix of foods to fuel our bodies and to keep them healthy. If the training load increases then extra food will also be needed to fuel the extra activity and to prevent fatigue.

A balanced diet containing appropriate amounts of carbohydrate, protein, fat, vitamins and minerals is the only way to achieve healthy eating and a rough guide would be to aim for 60% carbohydrate / 10-15% protein / and 25-30% fat in nutritional values of food. If you are a female aged between 19 and 50 years with a sedentary lifestyle, you will need around 2000 calories (2500 if male) each day to provide enough energy for everyday activities. A fast-food burger with fries and a milkshake would give you at least those 2000 calories so anything else that you eat that day becomes surplus to requirements. If this fast-food diet became the main food source you would quickly gain the calories but not the recommended daily nutritional values of vitamins and minerals which would lead to a feeling of tiredness and general ill health.

Make no sudden changes to diet or routine:

The horse's system needs routine so any dietary changes must be made very gradually and spread over several days to avoid problems.

What can *we* learn from this?

Changes to our own diet must also be made gradually. Our digestive system can easily be upset by introducing new foods that our stomach is not prepared to deal with e.g. increasing the amount of fibre in your diet may cause bloating and wind. Make changes over a period of time and your gut will soon adapt to accept the new levels.

Keep to the same daily feeding hours:

A horse who feels secure in his environment and in his daily routine is a happy horse. If you have a stabled horse you may already have experienced the sound of his hooves kicking the stable door in the morning because he knows it's breakfast time! Routine provides security but a regular feeding routine is also important to ensure that the 'little and often' rule can be adhered to throughout each day.

What can *we* learn from this?

We are all creatures of habit so routines can be both good and bad. A good habit would be getting into the routine of eating regular healthy meals; a bad habit would be getting into the routine of skipping breakfast every morning and then having a bag of crisps before lunch because you're hungry. Ask yourself this question; do you always eat because you are hungry or do you sometimes eat through habit or boredom?

Feed only good quality, clean forage:

Horses are naturally fussy eaters and will often turn up their noses if not given the best! Musty or dusty forage will affect condition and cause weight loss if not eaten. If eaten, it may even be harmful to their health.

What can *we* learn from this?

Don't be a dustbin! Eat fresh food whenever possible and avoid prepackaged convenience foods as these have little or no nutritional value. The manufacturing process generally destroys the natural vitamin and mineral content of food and large amounts of sugar, salt and artificial ingredients are often used to add colour and flavour.

Feed succulents daily:

In the case of the stabled horse, this is mainly to compensate for the loss of grass from the diet. Adding apples and carrots to feeds can also tempt fussy eaters.

What can *we* learn from this?

We need at least five portions of fruit and vegetables in our daily diet to ensure a healthy mix of nutrients. Many vitamins, minerals and antioxidants are found in fruits and vegetables and these are thought to play a large role in preventing coronary heart disease and cancer along with helping to fight infection by strengthening the immune system.

Allow at least one hour after feeding before exercising:

A full stomach will cause pressure on the diaphragm and lungs which will adversely affect the horse's breathing during exercise.

What can *we* learn from this?

The situation is the same in our own bodies. A full stomach will push against the diaphragm and create pressure on the lungs which will cause discomfort if our breathing rate goes up. Running around with a full stomach will usually result in an uncomfortable 'stitch' being felt.

Water before feeding:

Water is an essential part of the horse's diet and he should have a constant supply of fresh water available to him so that he can drink small amounts continuously throughout the day. Remember that the horse only has a small stomach so if he is denied water at any stage he will probably gulp down huge amounts when he is finally offered a drink and this would be problematic if he has just filled his stomach with a feed.

What can *we* learn from this?

Water is an essential part of our own diet too as around 60% of our body weight is water. Without it we would simply cease to function. Under normal circumstances, the body loses around two litres (three and a half pints) of water each day which must be replaced to prevent dehydration. The easiest way to do this is to drink water frequently throughout the day and it's important to be aware that coffee, tea and fizzy drinks that contain caffeine are all diuretics so cannot be used in place of water as they will actually take fluids away from the body. However, most vegetables contain 75-90% water so just keep eating those greens!

What have we learned?

The 'rules of feeding' we apply to our horses could certainly be applied to our own diets. Perhaps if we paid a little more attention to our own daily eating habits we ourselves could be feeling just as bright-eyed and bushy-tailed as our horses.

What, When, Why and How Much?

What should I eat? **When** should I eat it? **Why** should I eat it? **How much** of it should I eat?

Today's horse food manufacturers and their experts in equine nutrition have taken the hard work out of preparing the right mix of nutrients to feed to your horse by creating 'complete feeds' that cater for all stages of growth and development and are ready to use straight from the bag.

Horse owners strive to ensure that their charges receive the appropriate amount of good quality food to fuel their daily activities and to keep them in general good health and condition. We are all aware of the health risks associated with a horse becoming too thin or undernourished, the dangers of allowing a horse to become too fat and the potentially explosive hazards of a horse being over fed or inappropriately fed when not being exercised accordingly. Why then, as horse riders, do we pay such little attention to our own dietary requirements and the shape of our own bodies?

As stated earlier, a female of average weight with a fairly sedentary lifestyle will need around 2000 calories per day and a male 2500 to fuel everyday activities so a more active lifestyle – exercising regularly – will require more calories to fuel the extra activities and to prevent fatigue. The ideal daily balance of nutrients to achieve is around 60% carbohydrate, 10 – 15% protein, and no more than 25 – 30% fat with enough variety in the diet to ensure a healthy mix of vitamins, minerals, fluids and fibre. Bear in mind that although many common snack foods are high in energy-giving calories, these are provided mainly by sugar and fat so are not good sources of fuel as they don't provide a healthy balance of nutrients. For example, a small bag of crisps may contain as many as 200 calories but with a high fat and salt content; a small bar of chocolate may contain over 250 calories but with a 30% fat content; and a small can of fizzy drink contains around 145 calories, all provided by sugar alone.

Making sudden, dramatic changes to your diet is never advisable so plan to introduce healthier eating habits over a period of time. Your digestive system needs time to adjust to unfamiliar foods but gradual changes towards a healthier diet are also more likely to remain permanent. Abrupt, radical changes often lead to perceived withdrawal symptoms, rebellion and a big binge on everything you gave up!

Carbohydrates are the main energy providers so they are an essential part of every sports person's diet. They can be either 'simple' or 'complex' in form:

> • **Simple carbohydrates** – found in sweet tasting sugary foods such as cakes, biscuits and puddings
>
> • **Complex carbohydrates** – found in starchy foods such as bread, rice, pasta and potatoes

Both forms provide energy but simple carbohydrates create that instant 'boost' you feel when your blood sugar levels are raised. They are of limited use when it comes to fuelling your body for exercise as the effects are short lived and blood sugar levels soon drop again leaving you feeling tired. Complex carbohydrates provide a much slower release of energy so they keep you fuelled for activity throughout the entire day without the 'highs' and subsequent 'crashes' experienced when snacking on high sugar foods.

Carbohydrates are stored by the body in the liver and muscles in the form of glycogen. The supply must be regularly topped up as the depletion of glycogen stores is associated with tiredness and fatigue. Eating more complex carbohydrates and eating regularly helps to bolster the supply so gaps between meals should be no longer than four or five hours – eat little and often – to avoid hunger pangs and to prevent the potential for unhealthy snacking.

To keep up energy levels, an active individual with a busy working day followed by an hour or two of riding, muckling out etc. needs around 6 grams of carbohydrate per 1 kilogram of body weight per day to fuel their activities. Therefore, a person weighing 70 kilograms would need to consume 420 grams of carbohydrate daily (70 x 6g = 420g).

The amount of carbohydrate contained in packaged foods will be listed on the label with the total amount given and sometimes also the amount which is actually sugar. Choose items that have a high carbohydrate but low sugar content to ensure you gain the desired complex, rather than simple, carbohydrates. Non-packaged foods won't have any nutritional information stamped on them but fresh foods are always the healthier choice as highly processed, packaged foods will generally contain little or no food value. For this reason, whole-grain varieties of foods such as bread, rice and pasta will provide a more nutritious source of complex carbohydrates compared with white or 'quick cook' versions of the same as well as supplying a greater amount of fibre.

It can be particularly difficult to eat healthily when travelling to competitions. Burgers, chips and bacon butties are generally the main foods on offer and pre-competition nerves will often get in the way of eating anything at all! Remember the importance of keeping up those glycogen stores and continue to 'graze' throughout the day to keep your energy levels high. Listed below are some light meal and snack ideas that provide good sources of carbohydrate to keep you going all day and they can easily be prepared in advance and packed into your bag to take with you when you travel:

Snack Ideas: (approximate carbohydrate content given in brackets)

Source: *Energise For Exercise* by Penny Hunking.

- fruit and nut cereal bar (18g)
- large handful of raisins or dried fruit such as apricot, figs, dates (20g)
- small fruit scone (20g)
- apple, peach or pear (10g)
- banana (20g)
- satsuma (5g)
- toasted tea cake (30g)
- bagel (35g)
- currant bun or slice of fruit bread (20g)
- pot of low-fat yoghurt (25g)
- small tin or pot of low-fat rice pudding (40g)

Breakfast / Light Meal Ideas:

- glass of orange juice and a slice of toast (30g)
- two slices of toast and a boiled egg (30g)
- breakfast cereal with low-fat milk and a glass of fruit juice (30g)
- filled roll (wholemeal) – with low-fat filling such as tuna, salad, lean meat – and a small pot of yoghurt with fresh fruit (60g)
- tin of vegetable soup with two slices of wholemeal bread (60g)
- jacket potato with baked beans (60g)

You Can Take a Horse to Water...

Carbohydrates form only part of a balanced diet along with the other essential nutrients but your body cannot function at all without proper hydration. Just as your horse needs a plentiful supply of fresh water, your own body needs around two litres (three and a half pints) of water each day just to replenish the fluids used to keep all systems functioning as they should. It's not always easy to cope with the idea of drinking such a large amount of water every day so it's worth noting that many foods have a high water content which the body can make use of – most fruits and vegetables contain up to 90% water. It's also important to remember that tea, coffee, and most fizzy drinks don't count as fluids as they are all diuretics and will actually take water away from the body by increasing the amount of urine passed.

Water is obviously of equal importance to both the horse and the rider. Exercise creates heat and the body's response, whether equine or human, is to sweat in order to regulate the body temperature. Even exercising on a cold day raises the temperature enough to cause sweating so this fluid loss, along with the two litres (three and a half pints) already being used just to function, must be constantly replaced to prevent dehydration. A horse will continue to drink little and often throughout the day so that he remains well hydrated before, during and after exercise. The horse rider should learn from this example!

Dehydration, in either party, will very quickly cause a drop in performance and extreme dehydration causes many health problems ranging from muscle cramps and headaches through to organ failure and death, so it really is a matter of great importance and demands serious attention.

Checking your horse's hydration levels:

Your horse must always have fresh water available to him so an automatic trough is ideal – provided you can guarantee that it's used frequently – but water buckets are just as good if kept clean and topped up at all times. If you always find your horse's water bucket empty in the morning then he must be supplied with an additional bucket to prevent this from happening. An empty bucket may mean that he has been without water for some time and could already be dehydrated. Two simple ways to assess hydration levels are:

1. Check the colour of his urine and the consistency of his droppings

Urine should be plentiful and light in colour and droppings should be moist. Dehydration will cause urine to become dark in colour and droppings to become dry.

2. The skin pinch test

Take hold of a fold of skin (neck or shoulder) between your thumb and index finger and twist it gently left and right – without hurting the horse! – and then release it. The skin should snap back into place immediately if your horse is well hydrated. If there is a delay of over two seconds this indicates slight dehydration but if the delay is more than five seconds the horse is already heavily dehydrated. A horse can lose up to five litres (nearly nine pints) of body mass through sweat during intense exercise so without adequate hydration levels at the start of such sessions the horse will be placed under enormous stress and offering a bucket of water at the end of the session would then be too little too late!

Checking your own hydration levels:

Thirst is not a good indicator of needing to drink as by the time you feel thirsty you are already beginning to dehydrate. It takes only a 2% loss of body weight through dehydration to seriously affect your body's functions and a loss of 6% can become life threatening. Try weighing yourself before an exercise session and then again at the end to check your hydration levels. Each kilogram lost represents about one litre of fluid (each pound lost represents about 16 ounces of fluid). If you lose more than 1kg (2.2 lbs) during an exercise session there is a serious fluid deficit in your body which must be replaced as quickly as possible. Check your urine – it should be plentiful and pale yellow in colour. Dehydration will cause urine to become much darker, more scant and it may smell more strongly.

Easy Ways to Improve Hydration

The most effective way to remain well hydrated is simply to drink small amounts of water regularly. A horse will instinctively do this for himself, provided he has a constant supply available to him, but yet for ourselves this simple task often proves to be quite a challenge! We need to replenish the two litre (three and a half pint) deficit created by just existing so at least eight glasses of water are required each day. If you happen to have a water cooler at your workplace you will find that just sipping from a small cup on a regular basis soon adds up to the required amount without any concerted effort at all. Another hassle-free way to reach your daily target is to carry a refillable water bottle or sports bottle with you wherever you go and continue to drink frequently – little and often.

A lot of people struggle with this task because they don't like the taste of water. Many foods have a high water content so with a little thought it's possible to hydrate your body effectively in this way. The best choices are fresh fruit and vegetables as most contain at least 75% water:

- Grapes, oranges, apples, strawberries and bananas all contain between 75 – 90% water but melon contains the most at almost 95% water
- Carrots, watercress and tomatoes all contain around 90% water but lettuce tops them all with a content of over 95% water
- Low fat yoghurt, cottage cheese and skimmed milk also provide useful sources as all contain at least 80% water

Juice drinks and sports or energy drinks are another way to increase hydration levels but care must be taken when choosing this method. Many fruit juices and sports drinks are too concentrated to be absorbed easily by the body unless diluted so fluids are actually drawn from the body's existing water store to make use of them and this could cause dehydration! To make fruit juice less concentrated and to make water taste nicer simply mix the two together (half and half mix) to create your own juice drink. Sports drinks are available to buy in many different forms and they all promise to give you 'the edge' in competition. Unless you are facing many hours of intense effort without any food, the properties of such drinks are of little importance as the main concern is to remain suitably hydrated at all times. Check the label carefully to find the carbohydrate content. If it is higher than 8% (8g of carbohydrate per 100g of product) it will be difficult for the body to absorb and will therefore hinder hydration. If you are facing a long day of competition in particularly hot, sweaty weather you may benefit from the added mineral content of a sports drink but try making your own by using your home-made juice drink and simply adding a pinch of salt (just a few grains for every 100 ml ($3\frac{1}{2}$ fl oz) of fluid is sufficient) to the mixture.

Eat Well to Compete Well

You've done all the hard work. You've trained your horse and yourself in preparation for this big day. Don't undo all you've achieved by forgetting to eat and drink well on competition day!

The day before:
• Your body is fuelled today by what you ate yesterday, so what you eat today will be fuelling you tomorrow!
• Eat healthy, balanced meals with particular emphasis on complex carbohydrate content
• Eat little and often – keep gaps between meals to less than five hours
• Stay well hydrated by drinking suitable fluids or eating fresh fruits etc. throughout the day.

Competition day:
• Eat breakfast and then allow at least two hours for digestion before the event
• If you can't face breakfast, eat fruit or drink fruit juice at the very least as it will now have been more than five hours since your last meal and this will affect your glycogen stores
• Stay well hydrated by continuing to drink little and often
• Keep up your energy supplies by 'grazing' on high complex carbohydrate snacks or light meals at regular intervals
• On long-distance rides carry food and fluids with you at all times – top up whenever necessary – aim to drink regularly before you are thirsty and eat regularly before you are hungry!

CHAPTER FOURTEEN

Fun Ways to Keep Fit Through Riding

The aim of this book is to encourage riders of all abilities to get themselves as fit as their horse. The exercises used all target the specific muscle groups of most relevance to the rider and the routines focus on the areas of fitness training most needed in each equestrian discipline or the sport of riding in general.

Taking part in a sport you enjoy is a great way to get fit and then to keep fit. Improving your performance in your chosen sport through exercise provides a real incentive to stick with an exercise programme. For some, the decision to learn to ride in the first place may have come from nothing more than a desire to lead a more active life and now the only motivation they need to continue is the pure enjoyment of the sport.

Whatever your motivation, the rest of this chapter looks at some alternative equestrian sports that provide new challenges for all levels and, perhaps more importantly, a really fun approach to keeping fit.

BHS Trec:

BHS Trec can best be described as orienteering on horseback. Participants generally consider themselves to be equestrian tourists rather than competitors as it's scored by a points system and is not a race. Highly accessible to riders of all abilities it attracts everyone from the leisure rider through to the international competitor. The courses are designed to test the horse and rider through a range of activities combining the skills of trail riding, basic cross-country jumping and simple flatwork. Map-reading skills are needed but participants can take part in groups or in pairs as well as individually to help with the directions! Natural 'hazards' are included such as water crossings, riding under low branches, gates and obstacles that need to be tackled on foot.

Skills learned / Fitness gains:
- aerobic endurance
- flexibility
- balance / co-ordination

- map reading / knowledge of terrain
- access to beautiful countryside

Contact: The British Horse Society – http://www.bhs.org.uk

Horseball:

Horseball is a cross between rugby and basketball – played on horseback! To play horseball both horse and rider must be extremely fit as the game is played at high speed, mainly canter and gallop, for twenty minutes. The ball is slightly smaller than a football and has a harness over it to which are attached six handles. These handles allow the ball to be picked up off the ground (from the horse!) and passed to other riders. Played in teams, the ball must be passed from player to player at least three times before the team has the right to shoot at goal so good ball-handling skills are needed along with hand-eye coordination. Contact is permitted between players (this could be bodily contact between players or their horses) and the rules permit players to physically push each other off the playing field.

Skills learned / Fitness gains:
- aerobic endurance
- core strength / stability / balance
- flexibility
- hand-eye coordination
- fast, furious, competitive riding

Contact: The British Horseball Association – http://www.horseball.org.uk

---

Mounted Games:

Mounted Games (also known as gymkhana games) are a series of very fast races on horseback. Often considered to be a sport for children only, mounted games are actually open to riders of all ages although there is a height restriction for ponies of 148 cms (14.2 hands). Games can be in team, pair, or individual format and include races such as 'bending', 'sword lancers', or 'litter race' to name but a few. Designed to be accessible to all, no special equipment is needed and most ponies pick up the basics quickly.

Skills learned / Fitness gains:
- aerobic endurance
- core strength / stability / balance
- agility / flexibility

- hand-eye coordination
- team spirit / thrills and spills!

> **Contact:** The Mounted Games Association (GB) – http://www.mgagb.co.uk

Polocrosse:

Polocrosse is a combination of polo and lacrosse – on horseback.
Polocrosse is a team game but unlike polo only one horse is ridden per player for the duration of the match. Similar to lacrosse, the rider uses a stick to pick up the ball. The stick has a racquet-like head of loose net and the ball is made of sponge rubber. The object of the game is to score goals by throwing the ball between the opponent's goal posts.

Skills learned / Fitness gains:
- aerobic endurance
- core strength / stability / balance
- flexibility
- hand-eye coordination
- fast, tactical riding

> **Contact:** The United Kingdom Polocrosse Association–- http://www.polocrosse.org.uk

Vaulting:

Vaulting can best be described as gymnastics on a moving horse. Many people learn to ride through vaulting as the horse is controlled by a handler on the ground allowing the rider the opportunity to learn to move with the horse without the need to control the pace or the direction at the same time. Competitions exist for individuals and teams with as many as three riders sharing the same horse – at the same time!

Skills learned / Fitness gains:
- confidence
- balance / harmony with the horse
- strength / power
- flexibility / agility
- elegance / precision / graceful movement

> **Contact:** British Equestrian Vaulting – http://www.vaulting.org.uk

Carriage Driving:

Horse Driving Trials are based on eventing with each competition including three separate elements – dressage / marathon / obstacle driving. Many people try driving as a fun activity on holiday and then become hooked. Others have found that driving provides an opportunity to remain in contact with horses when riding is no longer an option. The fitness requirements vary depending on whether you choose to drive for pleasure or drive competitively but all levels certainly require mental agility.

Skills learned / Fitness gains:
- balance
- mental agility / coordination
- aerobic endurance (if walking courses for trials)
- flexibility / mobility (particularly if acting as 'groom' on the back!)

Contact: British Horse Driving Trials Association – http://www.horsedrivingtrials.co.uk

---

RDA Volunteer:

The Riding For The Disabled Association (RDA) provides an opportunity for disabled persons of all ages to try horse riding or carriage driving. The physical and psychological benefits of being around animals are many and the added opportunity to enjoy being outdoors can really promote a sense of well-being. Physiotherapists also believe that an hour spent on horseback, just moving with the movement of the horse, can replace many hours of conventional physiotherapy treatment. The RDA depends on volunteers to help run local groups and this provides an ideal opportunity to be around horses; to do something really worthwhile; and to keep fit. As a volunteer your main duties would include leading the horse or walking beside the horse to assist the rider with balance and control. This offers a great opportunity to enjoy a sociable hour in the company of others whilst exercising – a perfect way to keep fit!

Contact: Riding For The Disabled Association – http://www.rda.org.uk

---

Equercise™ – A Fitness Training Class for Riders

Many people find it difficult to remain motivated when exercising alone so joining an exercise class can often help to provide an incentive to stick with a regular routine. Equercise™ has been devised to bring together riders of all abilities in a fun, group environment to take part in riding specific exercises without the need to go to the gym or even leave the yard.

The circuit-style classes allow all participants to exercise together regardless of their current fitness level as everyone can work at their own individual pace. No special equipment is needed as only everyday yard items are used and an indoor or outdoor school provides an ideal venue. Below is an example of an Equercise™ class which was held in an indoor arena every Wednesday night for eight weeks during the winter months to help keep a group of mixed ability riders (and their non-riding friends) fit for the following competition season.

1. Warm up:
- Begin by walking around the edge of the arena at own pace until feeling warmer – music is a bonus if available
- While walking – shoulder shrugs and arm circles (Chapter Two)
- Change direction – heel kicks and knee lifts in walk (Chapter Five)
- Pick up the pace in the walk or try jogging for short intervals to elevate the heart rate or until a layer of clothing has to be removed!

2 Joint mobility exercises:
- Once warm – work through all of the joint mobility exercises detailed in Chapter Four to loosen and relax the body

3. Circuits – ten 'stations' set around the edge of the arena:
- Work in pairs (or small groups) and spread out around the arena
- Move in a clockwise direction spending one minute on each station

One – Side stretches
- Continue to alternate sides throughout (Chapter Two)

Two – Walk / jog
- Work at own pace – the challenge is to do the most laps in one minute!

Three – Hip swings
- Change legs after thirty seconds (Chapter Two)

Four - Side shuttles
- Skip for five strides in each direction before touching down (Chapter Six)

Five – Front lunges
- Alternate legs throughout and lunge with or without a bale (Chapter Six)

Six – Standing push-ups
- Use the edge of the arena or a lower platform (Chapter Seven)

Seven – Step-ups
• Use a bale or alternative step and work at own pace (Chapter Seven)

Eight – The plank
• Two people per bale (Chapter Five)

Nine – Travelling wide squats
• Squat five steps in each direction to keep moving (Chapter Five)

Ten – Abdominal crunches
• One person per bale – tummy tucks (Chapter Six) or cycle crunches (Chapter Nine)

4. Refreshment break:
• Continue to walk around slowly or keep feet gently on the move while taking a drink – take small sips to avoid a stitch.

5. Repeat circuits:
• Work in pairs as before
• Move in an anti-clockwise direction around the arena this time and spend only thirty seconds on each station (work faster?)

6. Cool down:
• Stay on the move by walking around the arena for around five minutes
• Gradually slow the pace as your heart rate and breathing rate recover

7. Stretches:
• Work through all of the daily stretches for upper body and lower body (Chapter Ten)
• Finish with the whole body stretch (Chapter Five)

Note: further details of Equercise™ classes can be found on http://www.equercise.com

Conclusion

This book began with the question, 'Are you as fit as your horse?' so it is perhaps appropriate to end with the question, 'Are you now prepared to do something about it if you are not?'

The contents of the book have highlighted the importance of fitness for the horse rider as well as the horse and the exercise plans have shown how easy it is to make big improvements to your fitness and flexibility for riding with just a little extra effort on a regular basis. It would be unrealistic of me to imagine that every suggested training programme is ideal for everyone and it's unlikely that any one routine will ever suit all individual circumstances but my intention has been to provide enough information, variety and scope to allow all riders to create an exercise plan that is specific to them; relevant to their sport; and, most important of all, fun to do!

The aim of this book has been to demonstrate how much can be done around the yard and within your existing routine to improve your fitness for riding without the need to take valuable time away from your chosen discipline. Think of an athlete training to perform in any sport – football, rugby, athletics, golf etc. – and you'll probably see an image of someone warming up by stretching and loosening their joints and perhaps even jogging in preparation. Think of a rider warming up and you'll probably see an image of someone sitting on a horse and riding around in circles. This may be preparing the horse but unless the rider has prepared his own body first, by working through some warm-up exercises before mounting, he is potentially stiff enough in the saddle to interfere with the horse's natural movement and this will result in the whole process taking much longer. Until all riders learn to appreciate their role as the human athlete working in partnership with the equine athlete, then this situation is unlikely to change. It is not considered 'normal' to warm up before mounting and it's 'not the done thing' to concentrate on rider fitness. It is perfectly normal to see a footballer warming up, so why not a rider? It is crucial for athletes in other sports to maintain or improve their fitness from one season to the next, so why not riders? Many areas of the horse world today are still governed by old traditions and many aspects of riding remain unchanged simply because we're told that 'It has always been done this way'. Change *can* be a good thing and I'll end this book with a tale that tells of the danger of getting stuck in our ways.

Tying Up the Cat

A long, long time ago there was a monastery in Japan. The abbot in charge was having a problem with an old alley cat who lived in the monastery garden and had taken to sitting on the wall each evening and yowling loudly during prayers.

After weeks of interruption the abbot could stand the yowling no longer and instructed a novice monk to tie up the cat each day before evening prayers. Cats being cats, this was no easy task and eventually just about every novice monk in the monastery became involved in the daily shenanigans of chasing down and tying up the cat.

A few years later the abbot died but the cat lived on and the monks continued to tie it up every evening before prayers. When the cat eventually died no one could actually remember why they had ever started tying it up in the first place but a new cat was brought into the monastery and dutifully tied up each evening – why break a tradition? Centuries later the ritual remained unchanged and members of the monastery began writing scholarly treatises about the religious significance of tying up a cat before evening prayers!

Now and again you will run into someone who insists that something must always be done in a certain way. If you ask that person *why* things must be done that way they will reply with, 'Because it's traditional'. Before following on blindly, stop and consider whether you are becoming the person who ties up the cat.

USEFUL CONTACTS

British Dressage Ltd.
Tel: 02476 698830
E-mail: office@britishdressage.co.uk
Website: http://www.britishdressage.co.uk

British Eventing
Tel: 02476 698856
E-mail: info@britisheventing.com
Website: http://www.britisheventing.com

British Horse Society (The)
Tel: 0870 1202244
E-mail: enquiry@bhs.org.uk
Website: http://www.bhs.org.uk

British Show Jumping Association
Tel: 02476 698800
E-mail: bsja@bsja.co.uk
Website: http://www.bsja.co.uk

Endurance GB
Tel: 02476 698863
E-mail: enquiries@endurancegb.co.uk
Website: http://www.endurancegb.co.uk

Equine Illustrations / Cartoons
Michael Musgrove – Studio Vert
Tel: 01902 343959

Equine Photography
John Steven
Tel: 01355 226524
E-mail: stevenequinepics@blueyonder.co.uk
Website: http://www.johnsteven.com

Peak Photography
Tel: 01501 770527
E-mail: harry@peakphoto.freeserve.co.uk
Website: http://www.peak-photography.co.uk

Equine Therapy

Equine Sports Massage Association
Haycroft Barn, Lower Wick, Dursley, Gloucestershire, GL11 6DD

Equine Sports Massage / Horsepower
Tel: 01651 869356 (Helen Tompkins)

Heart Rate Monitors
Bodycare Products
Tel: 01926 816155
E-mail: bcsales@lsi.co.uk
Website: http://www.bodycare.co.uk

Equine HRM -
http://www.horsehrm.com

Human HRM -
http://www.heartratemonitor.co.uk

Hurlingham Polo Association
Tel: 01367 242828
E-mail: enquiries@hpa-polo.co.uk
Website: http://www.hpa-polo.co.uk

Scottish Endurance Riding Club
Tel: 01835 863823
E-mail: lindsay.s.wilson@talk21.com
Website: http://www.scottishendurance.com

INDEX

abdominals, 12
adductors, 14
advanced drill four, 59
advanced hip swings exercise, 87
advanced stretches, 133–41
aerobic endurance, 5
anaerobic endurance, 6
ankles, 37
arm circles exercise, 19

back extensions exercise, 84
base fitness training, 15–23
    horse, 16–17
    rider, 17–23
BHS Trec, 172
biceps, 11
body composition, 7
    waist to hip ratio, 158
body stretch exercise, 50
bucking bronco exercise, 39

calves, 14
carriage driving, 175
cool down, 126–7
CRI Test, 147–8
cross-training, 150–1
cycle crunches exercise, 113

daily stretches, 127
    upper body, 127–8
    lower body, 128–9
dehydration, 168–70
dressage, 45–61
    dressage rider exercises, 50–5
dressage drills, 56–9

elbows, 36
elementary drill three, 58
endurance, 92–105
    endurance rider exercises, 96–103
Equercise™, 175–7
equine sports massage, 132–3
eventing, 74–91
    event rider exercises, 77–89

fat horse squats exercise, 40
fitness test
    walk test, 9
    run test, 156
flexibility, 7
forward seat squats exercise, 67
front lunges exercise, 66

girth tightener exercise, 99
gluteals (glutes), 13
grooming kit lifts exercise, 83

hamstrings, 13
heart rate monitor training
    horse, 145–8
    rider, 148–50
heels down exercise, 41
heel kicks exercise, 51
hip flexors, 13
hips/pelvis, 37
hip swings exercise, 20
hop overs exercise, 98
horseball, 173
hydration, 170–1

injury prevention
    complementary therapy, 132

jack knives exercise, 79
jockey squats exercise, 82
jumping circuit, 70–1

knees, 37
knee lifts exercise, 52

latissimus dorsi (lats), 12
leg at each corner exercise, 38
leg ups exercise, 97

Merrell® ten minute challenge, 9, 155,156
mounted games, 173

neck, 36
novice drill two, 57–8

obliques, 12
one and a half mile running test, 156

pectorals, 12
plank exercise, 55
polo, 106–18
    polo player exercises, 110–16
polocrosse, 174
posture stretch exercise, 86
power, 6
preliminary drill one, 57

quadriceps, 13

RDA volunteer, 175
rhomboids, 12

riding school, 31–44
    riding school rider exercises, 36–42
rules of feeding, 161

shoulder shrugs exercise, 18
show jumping, 62–73
    show jumping rider exercises, 65–70
side shuttles exercise, 68
side-step and squat exercise, 112
side stretches exercise, 20
sit and reach test, 10, 157
six-week training plan
    horse, 16–17
    rider, 17–23
smart goals, 144
speed, 6
standing push-ups exercise, 81
step-ups exercise, 78
strength, 6
stretches
    maintenance, 130
    developmental, 130
sumo squats exercise, 101
superman plank exercise, 100

torso toner exercise, 115
torso twist exercise, 88
travelling front lunges exercise, 55
travelling wide squats exercise, 52
triceps, 11
trunk rotation exercise, 22
trunk/spine, 37
tummy tucks exercise, 69
twister exercise, 102
twist and turn exercise, 110

vaulting, 174

waist to hip ratio, 158
warm-up, 122–3
    competition, 125–6
    routines, 123–5
wrists, 37